THE ENZYME ADVANTAGE

*For Health Care Providers
And People Who Care
About Their Health*

Also by Dr. Howard F. Loomis, Jr.

Enzymes: The Key to Health, Volume 1, The Fundamentals

THE ENZYME ADVANTAGE

*For Health Care Providers
And People Who Care
About Their Health*

By Howard F. Loomis, Jr., D.C., F.I.A.C.A.
with Arnold Mann

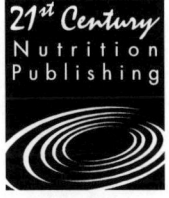

Copyright© 2015 by Dr. Howard F. Loomis, Jr.

Published by 21st Century Nutrition Publishing
800-662-2630

Without limiting the rights under copyright reserved above, no part of this publication may be reproduced, stored in, or introduced into a retrieval system, or transmitted, in any form or by any means (electronic, mechanical, photocopying, recording, or otherwise), without the prior written permission of both the copyright owner and the above publisher of this book. Excerpts or quotations are allowed for a book review.

Cover design, layout: Jessica R. Koman
Editor: Meredith H. Pond

Library of Congress Cataloging-in-Publication Data
Loomis, Howard F. Jr.
The Enzyme Advantage: for health care providers and
people who care about their health.
Includes selected bibliography and index.
1. Enzymes. 2. Nutrition. 3. Digestion. 4. Chiropractic.
Mann, Arnold.

First Edition, Printed in the USA

ISBN 978-0-9769124-1-5

DISCLAIMER: This book is not about treating disease, and no information contained in it should be construed as such. This book is about how food enzymes can be used to deliver nutrition, for the purpose of restoring normal function and maintaining health.

Acknowledgments

To **Arnold Mann** who asked me, "Do you have a book in you?" I've thoroughly enjoyed working with you as the book came to fruition, and we found that I did indeed have a book in me. Prior to this book, we shared one thing in common—great literature—you as a professional writer, researcher, and critic, and me as a fascinated reader. Thank you Arnold for articulating my work to the public with clarity, accuracy and eloquence.

To **Meredith Pond** for your editorial diligence. You are a consummate editor without whom many grammatical errors would have gone uncorrected.

To **Jessica Koman** for a design that is sure to enhance the reader's enjoyment of this book.

To **Laura Anne Sawall** for your undying dedication to seeing the project to its completion.

Dedication

For Christina and Howard,

Your births in the early 1970s not only changed my life, but refocused its direction as well. There was no doubt, in the years that would follow, you both would need me to be there for you. Through the years we have stayed close, and now you have your own beautiful families. In addition, you have allowed me to achieve my goals, and without each of you that would not have been possible.

Love, Dad

Table of Contents

Foreword—By Julie Penick, DNP, PhD, FNP-BC 1

Introduction 5

Part One—Recognizing Deficiency

Chapter 1—Desire 15

Chapter 2—Preparation 35

Chapter 3—Action 63

Part Two—What Is Your Deficiency?

Chapter 4—Carbohydrate: The Perfect Fuel 91

Chapter 5—Protein: The Body's Second Choice for Energy 113

Chapter 6—Lipid: The Last Resort 139

Epilogue—A Final Word 165

Selected Bibliography 169

Index 173

About the Authors 187

Foreword

By Julie Penick, DNP, PhD, FNP-BC

When I left bedside nursing to become a nurse practitioner, I quickly discovered that if I could not stretch myself beyond the allopathic model that I had been trained and educated in, there would be many people I would not be able to help. My desire to be of real service to people forced me into independent study of a wide range of health care and healing models.

In March of 2008, my studies led me to attend the Loomis Institute™ of Enzyme Nutrition: Seminar One. When I arrived home after the class, I told my husband, "that man [Dr. Loomis] is brilliant and as long as he is teaching I am going to attend every class he teaches." And while I haven't been able to attend *every* class Dr. Loomis has taught since then . . . I have come close!

You may be wondering what it was that I learned at that first seminar with Dr. Loomis that I found so remarkable. Through his clinical experience and his solid understanding of anatomy and physiology (structure and function), Dr. Loomis has developed the most comprehensive assessment approach I have ever studied. Use of his assessment model allows me to identify where an individual's stressors have interrupted homeostatic mechanisms. And since my interest has always been in restorative health care, I find Dr. Loomis's assessment model to be the most valuable tool I have when working with individuals.

Why do I say that?

Exposure to Dr. Loomis's triad approach resonated well with me. My Eureka moment came when I could overlay my triad "assessment lens" with Dr. Loomis's triad assessment model. For me, these triad domains lay the perfect foundation for assisting individuals in restoring or preserving their health.

The top of my triad assessment model is a circle with the diagnosis of "a body out of balance." Two circles, depicting the main reasons why the body lacks balance, make the base of my triad. These circles indicate that there is either a deficiency of something the body needs or there is an excess of something the body doesn't need. Dr. Loomis's assessment model was the first tool I had that allowed me to get greater information about those deficiencies and excesses.

Dr. Loomis's model insures that the individual is evaluated in both structure and function domains, while not ignoring the contribution of the Autonomic Nervous System. The model presents a triad platform for assessment that facilitates the ability to identify alterations from homeostasis and the contributing stressors that have resulted in the development of the individual's symptoms.

At the center of Dr. Loomis's assessment model is the identification of "stress points" that properly educated practitioners can access with their hands and assess. Identification of these "stress points" is solidly grounded in the basic sciences that all of the Healing Arts stand on. Add to that the ability to gain information about the condition of the extracellular fluid space through urinalysis testing, and you have a very comprehensive system of assessment.

The contribution of this sophisticated assessment model wasn't enough for this overachiever. Dr. Loomis continued his work developing a comprehensive "healing" approach by researching and developing food enzyme formulas that can provide the body with resources and support required to assist in overcoming the disruption of homeostasis. As you will read about in the book, oftentimes Dr. Loomis would use his own body as the research lab for food-enzyme formula testing!

I can honestly say that the thought of approaching an evaluation of an individual outside of the model Dr. Loomis has developed is to sell yourself and that individual short of all you have to offer.

With all the buzz talk in today's health care arena about "health promotion," there is no better way to approach this issue with individuals than with the application of Dr. Loomis's assessment model and health restoration approaches. That is, of course, my opinion—humble or not.

I want to leave you with this one thought that I have "borrowed" from Dr. Loomis. Your professional training program taught you the skills you need to be a competent practitioner. The journey to becoming a healer is your responsibility!

Introduction

Medicine will always be in search of the magic bullet—that pill or potion that will do exactly what it was intended to do, and *only* what it was intended to do, every time, for every patient.

This is the Holy Grail of modern medicine.

The problem is, it doesn't exist!

It doesn't exist because no two individuals are identical, because biochemical circumstances will vary from time to time and over time, and because organs and organ systems other than those targeted will inevitably be affected. The proton pump inhibitor—designed to shut down the production of stomach acid (HCl) and give an irritated esophageal lining time to heal—will also impair protein digestion and fat digestion. How?

For protein, the pump shuts down the conversion of pepsinogen into to pepsin. For fat, the pump stems the flow of bile, which is stimulated by the production of stomach acid.

These and more serious side effects have led to a resurgence of interest in alternative/natural approaches. And it isn't just about drugs. It's about what has been described as a change in thinking on the part of practitioners—a shift from the original inductive mindset, of conducting a *complete and thorough* examination and looking at all the evidence—to a more deductive, formulaic approach to diagnosis and treatment.

One of the earliest voices lamenting this shift in thinking was the 19th century English physician Thomas Addison. Addison was one of medicine's greatest diagnosticians. To his credit is Addison's disease, a skin condition resulting from the progressive destruction of the adrenal glands. A host of other disorders includes Addisonian anemia, which is now known as pernicious anemia, resulting from Vitamin B12 deficiency; and, Addison-Schilder syndrome, a metabolic disorder also known as Adrenoleukodystrophy. Addison is also credited with discovering the pathology of pneumonia.

But the greatest contribution to medicine during his time, Addison declared, was René Laennec's stethoscope, which "contributed more towards the advancement of the medical art than any other single individual, either of ancient or modern times."

Addison loved Laennec's stethoscope. And yet, he had harsh words for the way medicine had come to depend on it, at the expense of physical diagnosis. Addison, who would sit at a patient's bedside and use all of his senses, all of his intellect, all of his powers of physical sensation and observation to tease out a diagnosis inductively, came to deplore the arrival of what he called the "stethoscopist."

"The enthusiasm, the rashness, the bigotry and conceit of the exclusive stethoscopist," he wrote, "have indeed, most seriously retarded the adoption, and vitiated the claims of physical diagnosis. ... They seem to look upon the instrument as all-sufficient; they rush at once to auscultation and percussion; they neglect or disdain to make those careful and minute inquiries, which no sound and sensible physician ever fails to do, and thereby convert an invaluable auxiliary into what, in their hands at least, proves but an imperfect and treacherous substitute."

And so the world of deductive medical thinking entered, listening through the stethoscope to the heart, the lungs and the bowels for the sound that would dictate the treatment, rather than taking a complete history and performing a hands-on physical exam, using all one's senses and investigative powers to build a diagnosis inductively based on what the body as a whole was saying at that moment.

Introduction

As a young student at Logan College of Chiropractic, in the late 1960s, I was unable to use the stethoscope because of a hearing impairment from childhood. In order for me to pass the clinical examination and start seeing patients, the Logan clinicians taught me how to evaluate a patient's pulse pressure and pulse rate with my hands. I was also taught how to distinguish between a stroke patient and a heart attack patient with my hands when the patient was unconscious, and to detect lung problems by placing my fingers between a patient's ribs and having them take deep breaths while I felt for any telltale vibration.

I was learning to diagnose with my hands and to think inductively.

Of particular interest to me was a book called *Clinical Judgment,* by Alvin Feinstein (The Williams & Wilkins Co., 1967), which showed how to sort through the evidence and, by way of inductive thinking, evaluate which piece or pieces of evidence were most revealing, and then make the diagnosis.

Arthur Conan Doyle, a physician himself, modeled the great Sherlock Holmes after his renowned mentor and anatomy professor, Dr. Joseph Bell, known for his fastidious attention to detail. Dr. Bell taught his students to use all of their senses, especially their powers of observation, in making a diagnosis.

And so Doyle's character, Sherlock Holmes, the great detective, weighed every piece of evidence leading to each "elementary" observation, and finally his ultimate "diagnosis" as to *who done it.*

So, is medicine becoming a lost art in pursuit of formulaic thinking? A good question.

In their 1963 book, *Physical Diagnosis: The History and Examination of the Patient,* authors John Prior and Jack Silberstein lament the fact that little space is given to the case history in textbooks on physical diagnosis and the development of the medical examination. In their opinion, a diagnostician wasn't worth anything if he or she could not take a correct and thorough case history and do a good examination.

And they were right. A thorough case history and physical exam is absolutely necessary if one is to detect deviations from normal, which should be at the heart of any diagnostic process.

It was right around this time, while I was at Logan College, that I read Hans Selye's landmark book, *The Stress of Life*, which demonstrated the role of stress in the development of disease. He said that the early symptoms of any condition are vague and nondescript, so that one cannot really know what is going on until an actual disease can be diagnosed.

For Selye, this progression to disease involved a lack of adequate nutrition, suggesting that providing the right nutrition would be a good strategy for halting the progression to full-blown disease.

This made perfect sense to me, because I knew that my chiropractic career would not be spent diagnosing diseases. But if one can detect early deviations from normal—by conducting a thorough patient history, including diet, and a thorough hands-on examination, and blood and urine testing—these early deviations should be correctable by providing the right nutrition to restore normal function, and possibly halting the progression to the disease state.

It all seemed quite elementary, in principle. Instead of masking symptoms with medications, why not provide the body with the nutrition it needs to heal the underlying problem itself?

Such a strategy would in fact be urged in a 2001 editorial in the *Journal of Postgraduate Medicine*, entitled "The Case for an Ancient Cause."

Introduction

In it, the authors note that the ancient Greeks believed that Asclepios, the god of medicine, had two daughters—one responsible for prevention, the other for cure. Hippocrates, the father of Western medicine, was an inductive thinker and forceful advocate for prevention. The authors note that Hippocrates urged physicians "to pay attention to the environmental, behavioral, and social context in which illness occurs." His exact words: To consider the "mode of life of the inhabitants, whether they are heavy drinkers, taking lunch, and inactive, or industrious, eating lunch, and drinking little."

"Have we heeded this Hippocratic challenge?" The authors ask. "Do we favor one daughter of Asclepios at the expense of the other?" It's all a matter of maintaining health and preventing disease, as opposed to simply treating the symptoms with drugs and dealing with the full-blown disease when it appears.

It's the difference between a health care system and a sick care system.

Hence, the growing interest on the part of patients in so-called alternative health care practitioners for concerns such as back pain, digestive disorders, arthritis, sprains and strains, allergies, high blood pressure, headaches, insomnia, chronic immune problems, and anxiety and depression.

What do all of these conditions have in common? They are all primarily symptomatic, with an absence of concrete pathology to say *where* the conditions are coming from.

For 12 years after graduating from Logan College, I did my inductive best to come up with a method, a system, to restore normal function and maintain health. Along with my physical exam, my blood work and urinalysis, I experimented with every nutritional supplement available—protein supplements, carbohydrates, lipids, vitamins, minerals, you name it—in an effort to discover dependable strategies for relieving my patients' symptoms and slowing their progression to disease. One of the things working against me was the fact that nutritional deficiencies usually don't become apparent for 60 to 90 days; and when they do, the symptoms are vague and overlapping.

In the end, nothing works, not with any real consistency.

Then along came Dr. Edward Howell and his enzymes.

If indeed a magic bullet existed, one that could be tapped for medical purposes, it would be the enzyme. Howell himself called them Nature's Workers—each created by body cells to do one job and one job only, with a consistency dating back to the beginning of time.

Three such enzymes, central to Howell's work *and* this book, are the digestive enzymes amylase, protease and lipase, which digest carbohydrates, proteins and fats, respectively, so that they may be absorbed and used by the body as building blocks and fuel. Then there are the food enzymes, as Howell called them, which exist in all living things, plant and animal, and which facilitate their own life functions and assist in their digestion when they are consumed as food by another organism.

And so the lipase contained in whale blubber assists in its digestion when it is consumed by the Eskimo, or protease enzymes contained in various meats, cellulase in fruits and vegetables, and so on.

It's all part of Nature's cycle of life.

Unfortunately, as Dr. Howell discovered back in the 1920s, with the advent of cooking, pasteurizing and processing, the enzymes contained in the foods we eat have been destroyed, compromising our ability to digest them completely. The result is incomplete digestion leading to nutritional and energy deficits as body organs struggle to

Introduction

do their part in maintaining health, and, ultimately, progression to the degenerative diseases—from arthritis and diabetes to heart disease and cancer.

It is this progression from health to disease that concerns this book, with supplemental enzymes as a means of achieving more complete digestion and providing the nutritional elements needed for body cells to maintain normal function *and* reducing an individual's risk of progression to the degenerative diseases.

During the following five years, from the time I met Howell, I would develop just such a system for diagnosing nutritional deficiencies in various organ systems and using food enzyme supplements to deliver the specific nutrition needed to the struggling organ system to restore normal function, and health.

Starting with my own ears.

Dr. Howard F. Loomis, Jr.
Madison, Wisconsin, April 2015

Part One—Recognizing Deficiency

Your body requires food to produce energy. It prefers carbohydrates, but can convert protein when needed to make up for a temporary drop in energy. The problem is that protein is needed for growth and repair of tissues, and a multitude of other functions. The use of protein for energy is responsible for many types of symptoms and especially cravings.

Chapter 1

Desire

The first time young Anthony Collier came to my chiropractic office in Forsyth, Missouri, in 1980, I didn't want anything to do with the digestive enzyme supplements he was trying to introduce to health care providers.

During the past 12 years, from the day I first hung out my shingle in May 1968, I had done everything I could to make nutritional supplements useful in my practice. But in terms of relieving a patient's symptoms, I couldn't find any consistent pattern of benefit from any of them—except for digestive symptoms. Occasionally, I would send patients with digestive problems next door to Tony Collier's offices to buy digestive enzymes. But, I just couldn't see any broader way of incorporating them into my practice.

Or so I thought. I had no idea that Tony Collier's visit to my office that day would turn out to be a life-changing moment for me, in every way imaginable.

Collier had recently relocated the National Enzyme Company, founded by Dr. Edward Howell in 1932 as a small mail-order operation, to the Civil War-era town of Forsyth, a winding drive east through the Ozarks from the "micropolitan" music mecca that is Branson, Missouri. He had bought the entire complex next door and was setting up manufacturing, and what he hoped would be national and ultimately global sales.

Dr. Howell's Theory

Dr. Howell's involvement in digestive enzyme supplements had grown out of his early discovery that the natural enzymes contained in the foods we eat, which Nature intended to assist us in our digestion of these foods, are destroyed during the cooking process, and during pasteurization.

Basically, heat kills these "food enzymes."

This, Howell theorized, places a larger than normal burden on the human pancreas to produce enough enzymes to digest everything in our enzyme-deficient cooked and processed food diet. Destroyed are the protease enzymes that digest protein, lipases that digest fats, and amylases that digest starches.

The inability of the human pancreas to fully meet this demand, Howell wrote in *Enzyme Nutrition: The Food Enzyme Concept*, results in the accumulation and putrefaction of partially digested foods in the large and small intestines, and an inflammatory cascade responsible for many of the chronic diseases afflicting humankind today—from arthritis and diabetes to heart disease and cancer.

In contrast, these widespread chronic diseases are not commonly found among carnivores and herbivores that live in the wild and eat enzyme-rich raw foods, as Nature originally intended.

That was Howell's theory.

And that's what led him to digestive enzyme supplements as a means of replacing the missing food enzymes in the human diet and achieving more complete digestion. Actually, the more appropriate term here is *predigestion*, because food enzymes, from raw foods or from food enzyme supplements, do their digestive work in the upper part of the stomach, or the "food enzyme stomach," as Howell called it. That's before the food we eat is acted upon by protein-digesting pepsin in the lower stomach, and pancreatic enzymes in the small intestine.

And that's the message that Collier was trying to deliver to the health care establishment in 1980, with the hope that his enzyme supplements would find a more broad clinical application in the hands of the right practitioners, myself included.

But the dozen years leading up to Collier's arrival at my door were filled with nothing but disappointment, even though I started out in my practice convinced that vitamin and mineral supplements, in combination with pancreatin (animal enzymes), would prove a breakthrough in dealing with the more difficult-to-treat, visceral aspects of chiropractic care.

Twelve Long Years

Chiropractic, as originally conceived and taught, doesn't *only* deal with structure and with manipulation techniques meant to restore proper alignment and relieve stress and its resulting pain.

In chiropractic, you get the same basic education over a five-year period that a medical doctor gets—anatomy, physiology, biochemistry, pathology, microbiology, radiation, and so on.

The difference is, the medical doctor then goes after drug therapy and function, and the chiropractor goes after structure.

Or that's the way chiropractic has come to be perceived, as dealing exclusively with structure.

In fact, that's only half the equation. Structural misalignment is but one source of stress and pain, and one aspect of traditional chiropractic care.

When a person comes to see a chiropractor with pain in the shoulder, lower back or neck, that pain may actually be the result of stress caused by an organ system dysfunction—gallbladder, stomach, lung, etc.

That's the visceral side of chiropractic, and it's inextricably linked to the structural side, from the day we are conceived and begin to develop in the womb until the day we die. It is pure yin and yang. And it's often impossible to sort out in terms of exactly where in the body an individual patient's symptoms are located. It could be an alignment problem, or it could be organ dysfunction due to nutritional deficiency. It's a domino effect that is causing the stress that is causing the involuntary muscle contraction that is causing the misalignment that is resulting in pain.

A good example is scurvy.

Chapter 1—Desire

Before Deficiencies Become Apparent

Most of us know scurvy as a disease of long-ago sailors whose voyages around the world without citrus left them vitamin C deficient, with their gums bleeding and their teeth falling out. Libraries are full of the accounts of sea captains losing their crews back in the 1600s and 1700s, before it was discovered that fresh citrus was insurance against this scourge.

Scurvy always started the same way.

First, the crew member became tired. Then his joints became stiff and sore as he tended to his duties aboard the ship. Then his gums became pink and spongy, with bleeding from the mucous membranes. He would break out in little red blotches, hemorrhages on his skin, usually on his thighs and legs. Finally, his teeth would start falling out, followed by jaundice, neuropathy, fever, convulsions and ultimately death.

All of this disappeared with the discovery that a vitamin C deficiency was behind scurvy. Or did it disappear? In fact, scurvy still exists in society today on a more subliminal level. People who are vitamin C deficient complain of being tired. "I can hardly get out of bed," they say. And yes, they may suffer from bone pain.

But these days, it's not diagnosed as scurvy; it doesn't reach that advanced stage of symptoms because we have better diets. The same is true of other vitamin- and mineral-deficiency disorders, which rarely reach full bloom. Examples include beriberi (B1), pellagra (B3), and rickets (D). They're not diagnosed, but the early symptoms are still there, emanating from nutritionally deprived organ systems.

A diagnosis can get pretty complicated.

Vitamin C is part of the protein cascade. Water soluble vitamins B and C fit into carbohydrate metabolism. Vitamin C and sulfur are specific for protein. And vitamins A, D and E are all fat soluble vitamins. In the end, everything's connected to deficiencies and overlapping symptoms.

And so the idea came to me, while I was a chiropractic student at Logan College of Chiropractic: Dietary supplements might prove to be an effective means of dealing with the more difficult visceral aspect of chiropractic care, *if* I could figure out which supplements to use in specific situations.

On graduation, I chose what I thought would be a good starting point.

I knew I would be seeing a lot of patients with intervertebral disc degeneration.

Food *for* Thought

Intervertebral discs, which provide shock absorption and range of motion for the spine, are like old-fashioned golf balls. The outside plastic covering of the golf ball corresponds to the ligaments that hold the disc between the vertebrae. The coil of rubber bands under the ball's covering corresponds to the next layer down, the disc annulus, which is made of collagen. The annulus stabilizes and works in concert with the disc nucleus to equalize pressure and prevent damage from stress to the vertebrae. Like the liquid center of the golf ball, the disc nucleus contains a jelly-like liquid. Besides acting as a shock absorber, the disc-nucleus keeps our vertebrae separated, so they can rotate freely on one another as we turn to see who is coming our way, or as we pivot to strike a golf ball.

Now to my strategy.

The liquid at the center of these intervertebral discs is made up of a mixture of water and protein. It's the protein that holds the water in place, in jelly-like suspension, and maintains the integrity of the nucleus. Without protein, the water would leak out of the nucleus, the disc would thin, and the patient would experience stress, pain, and loss of flexibility in the spine.

Thus, I reasoned that patients with thinned-out discs may be having a problem with protein metabolism.

It made perfect sense.

And so I emerged from my chiropractic training wanting to improve protein digestion and metabolism in my patients who had low back problems. That was my opening foray into this nutritional approach.

I had at my disposal many nutritional supplements. One was Betaine HCl. Betaine is a protein derived from the beet root. The HCl, which stands for hydrochloride, is a salt used by the pharmaceutical industry to get drugs absorbed across the gut wall.

So I had HCl to improve assimilation. The Betaine also helps the liver metabolize protein once you've digested it.

Then there were the protein supplements. Spirulina was a very good one.

I also used a supplement called ox bile salts to help improve the flow of bile, to aid in the breaking down of fats and the absorption of vitamins A, D, E and K.

And I had the pancreatic enzymes, pancreatin, that I thought facilitated more complete digestion of protein.

I was going to be the 90-day wonder. I had my Betaine HCl, I had ox bile salts, I had my protein supplements, and I had pancreatin to help protein digestion.

Those were my tools. I was ready to go.

I had been trained in laboratory work at Logan, in blood and urinalysis. Furthermore, I had written a urinalysis program that would tell me when the patient wasn't digesting protein and how it was affecting the body. I was set to go.

Unfortunately, the bottom line was that I could never get any improvement in the tests. There was no detectible improvement in protein assimilation. The protein wasn't being properly digested. And I wasn't getting any significant improvement in joint range of motion in the spines of my patients.

That was just one approach. Over the next 12 years, I used everything under the kitchen sink—all manner of supplements, including vitamins and minerals, and manipulating people's diets, you name it. Nothing worked.

No objective signs appeared that I could measure to know *every time* when to give what—not urinalysis or blood tests or physical examination—none increased range of motion or loss of muscle contraction. I was checking everything under the sun, and no matter what supplement I was using, I could find no consistent, reliable benefit for any symptom or cluster of symptoms.

Something in my equation was clearly missing. I could adjust and get relief for my patients, but too often the relief wouldn't last, because the source of the pain was visceral, not structural. And I couldn't make a dent in the visceral aspect with nutritional supplements.

This went on for more than a decade.

Right up to the day that Collier showed up with his digestive enzyme supplements. He took me to lunch. A nice young man, he obviously believed in his product. I just didn't see any reason to pursue it any further than I already had. To make matters worse, the

Chapter 1—Desire

infections in my ears were draining and making me miserable that day, as they had been for the past 43 years.

The Doctor Becomes The Patient

It's been said, if you want to motivate a doctor, give him a disease.

I was 10 months old in 1938 when an attack of whooping cough took away half my hearing.

My mother never forgave the doctor.

"That's nonsense," he had said over the phone. "You're a new mother, you're a nurse, and you're imagining things. The child doesn't have whooping cough. I'll come by and check on him if he isn't feeling better by Monday."

We were living in the small town of Dunkirk, on the banks of Lake Erie in western New York. By Monday, when the doctor showed up at our house with his own son, as my mother recalled, he took one look at me, turned white as a sheet, grabbed his son, and ran out the door without so much as a word.

My mother never allowed him in our house again.

Whooping cough, or pertussis, was a terror back in 1938. Caused by the highly contagious bacteria Bordatella pertussis, it typically starts off with mild symptoms that gradually develop into severe coughing fits of five to 10 forceful coughs, marked by the high-pitched "whoop" sound as the infant or child inhales air after coughing. The coughing stage of the disease usually lasts about six weeks before subsiding. In some cases, the child does not survive.

My mother and my father's mother, both nurses, cared for me, giving me the gold shots the doctor ordered. Penicillin wouldn't be introduced until after World War II, although the best that antibiotics would ever offer in the case of active whooping cough would be to shorten the infectious stage of the disease.

I was quarantined. My father, the town baker and family bread winner, was forbidden to enter my room.

There were times when my mother did not expect me to live.

I did survive. But those big whoops can cause a lot of problems, including bleeding from the blood vessels in the eyes, rib fractures, fainting, urinary incontinence, hernias—and yes, bilateral hearing loss.

That's what I was left with. The severity of the cough knocked out my hearing in both ears, like a hurricane wiping out two neighboring towns. Depending on whether it was winter or summer, I would test between 40 percent and 50 percent of normal hearing range. And the early language sounds I'd started making at 10 months old stopped, my mother said. I didn't say another word until I was three years old.

Worse for me were the constant ear infections and the excruciating earaches that went with them. Both of my ears were continuously draining pus from middle ear infections that neither my immune system nor any antibiotic could touch. I would spend weeks lying in bed, my ears throbbing with pain. I missed a half year of school every year with those infections.

When I was age 13, I had my tonsils out, and the worst of those earaches disappeared. But the infections remained as a continuous, purulent draining out of both ears, which is why I was not able to wear a hearing aid. Nothing could go inside my ears because of those infections.

My hearing loss persisted.

The only thing that saved me in school was that I could read. This came from my early interest in sports, starting with my listening to

Chapter 1—Desire

late-night boxing matches on the family radio inside one of those big consoles. I would lie on the floor and sink my teeth gently into the molding along the bottom of the cabinet. I could hear, because of the bone conduction. The first fight I remember was when Billy Conn came back to fight Joe Lewis in their 1946 rematch. I was eight years old, and I became a huge boxing fan. The next morning I would read about the fight in the sports section of the newspaper. Then came basketball.

So I learned to read the sports section. I also had a huge collection of baseball cards and could recite every statistic on the back of every player's card.

I still couldn't hear, though. My teachers had little patience with me because I seemed to be off in my own world. Then, my sixth grade teacher, Mrs. Clark, realized how well I could read and introduced me to the library.

The first thing she showed me was the dictionary. "You should be able to open this book and put your finger right where the 'Q' is," she told me. So I made friends with the dictionary, and then the encyclopedia.

Finally, she took me to the card catalogue and taught me the Dewey Decimal System, and how all the books were arranged.

I owned the library after that. I was reading Carl Sandburg's *Life of Lincoln* that summer.

That book set me up for the rest of my life.

My big break on the hearing front came in 1958 when I learned about the bone conduction hearing aid. Unlike conventional hearing aids, which go inside the ear and provide amplification of sound for people with hearing loss due to nerve damage, this hearing aid fit on a pair of glasses and pressed up against the bone behind the ear for people like me with conduction hearing loss. With the hearing aid, it was like listening to the boxing matches on my parents' radio again, but instead of the sound being transmitted into my inner ear through my teeth, it was being transmitted clearly through the bones behind my ears.

When my hearing was tested, it came out at 110 percent. I couldn't believe the noise!

And so my hearing life began, though the chronic, draining, ear infections persisted. The only thing that ever helped was the antibacterial drug Gantrisin, approved in 1950. I still remember the afternoon visits to Dr. Rosten. The standard oral dose did nothing. Then he gave me a shot in my buttocks. That didn't work. Finally, he gave me a double shot in the buttocks along with the oral dose, and that did the job. The ear infection stopped. But as soon as I mowed the lawn, or got any water in my ears at all, the infection returned.

So I continued living most of the time with my draining ears. But from age 20, I could hear!

I wound up taking night classes at the University of Buffalo and working days at Dunlop, in the mailroom. Then, the company put me on the road as an auditor, counting tires in its warehouses. One of four such auditors, I covered the Midwest region, from Portland, Maine, to Albuquerque, New Mexico.

The last thing I was thinking of back then was becoming a chiropractor. I had watched my father become one, and I wanted nothing of it. In 1948, he had a terrible auto accident resulting in a low back injury that plagued him for several years. He had to give up his profession as a baker.

The only medical person to put him back on his feet was a local chiropractor. So my father became a chiropractor. He graduated from Logan College of Chiropractic in 1955, the same year I graduated

Chapter 1—Desire

from high school. This work gave him a new life. But all I remember from those years was the financial hardship my family endured while he was unable to work. As he made his way through Logan, we lived in a rundown triplex, and we scraped by in the years that followed as he struggled to build his practice.

I wanted no part of this life as a chiropractor.

That all changed, however, when I was in Des Moines one week doing an audit and I ran into the assistant dean at Palmer College, who was in town to raise money and talk to students and local practitioners. He invited me along to see a side of chiropractic I'd never seen before—nice homes and nice offices.

And I remembered the only person who helped me with my ears when I was growing up was a chiropractor. He'd adjust me with what was called the basic technique. He'd lie me face down and get his thumb under the bottom part of my sacrum, the tail bone, and he'd elevate me as he went up my spine, manipulating every bone, looking for muscle contraction and subluxation, which happens when one or more of the bones of the spine move out of position and create pressure on or irritate the spinal nerves. It worked every time. It slowed down the drainage and some of the inflammation, and my hearing improved.

Chiropractic was the only thing that ever helped me, besides the Gantrisin shots.

I knew I didn't want to spend the rest of my life counting tires. So I called the Dean at Logan, who remembered my father. The next week I called my boss at Dunlop and told him I was leaving to start school the next month in St. Louis.

At Logan, the day I walked in, I knew I was home. I've been in love with chiropractic from day one. It's all about the science. It's been a never-ending challenge, with a life-altering payoff for me that began when Tony Collier came to visit in 1980.

Another Try

As I said, the day Collier arrived at my door, I was convinced that his enzyme supplements would be of no benefit to my patients, beyond relieving their digestive symptoms. Years of beating my head against the supplement wall had convinced me.

And yet, something Tony's brother had given me started me thinking.

It was a new edition of Dr. Howell's first book, *Food Enzymes for Health and Longevity*. In the Foreword to the revised 1980 edition, Viktoras Kulvinskas described a phenomenon called "leukocytosis," whereby there is an "excessive augment of white blood corpuscles in the blood." This increase in white blood cells usually occurs when the body is fighting infection or during an allergic reaction. However, the white blood cell count can also go up after strenuous exercise, as a result of emotional stress, or during pregnancy or labor.

And leukocytosis also can occur during digestion.

The German physician Rudolph Carl Virchow was the first to describe "digestive leukocytosis," though he saw nothing to be concerned about, since the white blood cell counts went up every time his study participants ate a meal.

Dr. Paul Kouchakoff stunned the First International Congress of Microbiology in Paris in 1930 by presenting his findings from thousands of blood samples taken after people had eaten three different types of foods:

1. Natural raw foods, such as fresh vegetables, nuts, raw honey, raw eggs, raw meat, raw fish
2. Cooked foods
3. Manufactured foods—products such as sugar, wine, vinegar and chocolate.

There was no jump in the white blood cells with the natural, uncooked, raw foods, but there was leukocytosis with the cooked foods—as if a virus or bacteria had entered the body. Factory-produced foods also caused a jump in white blood cells, especially wine, sugar and vinegar.

Cooked, smoked and salted animal flesh brought the biggest jump in white blood cells.

Leukocytosis occurred as early as 3 to 5 minutes after eating began, typically peaked at 30 minutes, and the counts returned to normal by 90 minutes.

I remember sitting in my living room reading about this. My pet boxer, Gussie, was sitting nearby. I read about the absence of food enzymes in the cooked foods we eat and how the immune system has to send in white blood cells, which are loaded with enzymes, to assist in digestion. Instant leukocytosis.

That's when it hit me. I literally jumped out of my seat and yelled "Yes," scaring the hell out of poor Gussie. "Now I know why the supplements don't work. They're not getting digested, and we're taxing the immune system!"

Suddenly I could trace the chronic immune problems my patients were experiencing to incomplete digestion. The immune system wasn't being called on to assist in digestion; it was being called on to deal with all the toxic garbage that wasn't being digested. And it had to do this every time we ate a meal. It was an enormous tax on the immune system which, as a result, had problems fulfilling its primary duties—fighting off infections.

The next time Collier came by, he brought his chemist with him. He knew I did blood and urine testing, and he was eager to get me involved. But I still wasn't sure about the enzyme supplements, or how to use them. What I needed to know first was how to determine if a patient was deficient in a particular enzyme.

What are the signs of a protease deficiency? I asked. Neither Collier nor his chemist knew. Collier suggested I call Dr. Howell, who by then was in his 80s and retired in Florida. I had my note pad ready when I got him on the phone. *But he didn't know either.*

Nobody had ever looked for signs of specific enzyme deficiencies.

So how would you know when to use them?

I decided to experiment with the broad product they were selling—a capsulized blend of plant-derived enzymes with protease, lipase, maltase and cellulase.

I had tried this blend before, and it hadn't done much of anything. It didn't improve digestion enough, it didn't change urinalysis, it didn't change the blood tests enough. I figured maybe it wasn't strong enough. I asked Tony to increase the potency of the blend. The technology to make enzyme preparations stronger, or increase their catalytic "activity levels," had just come about.

They boosted the activity level of the blend and made me 100 bottles, which I gave to 100 patients, asking them to take two capsules with each meal for 30 days. I did extensive case histories and chiropractic examinations. Patients had a variety of problems, primarily structural, such as joint pain, back pain, elbow pain,

Chapter 1—Desire

headaches, digestive problems, and so on. Nothing in the actual disease realm.

One Enzyme At A Time

My hope was that when patients came back I would be able to deduce from examinations, and blood and urine tests how to use these enzymes. There was no common denominator. But patients said they felt so much better, they could digest their food better, and they slept better. They all wanted more. But I didn't know how the enzyme blend worked. One size doesn't fit all. What would I do with it? Give it to everybody?

That's when I decided to take a different course of action.

"What we have to do," I told Collier, "is isolate each individual enzyme and study it by itself. Let's take pure doses of protease, pure doses of lipase, and study them one enzyme at a time."

I had a special interest in protein, so we started with the protease enzyme.

Once again I told Tony to concentrate it; make it stronger than it was in the original digestive formula.

"I don't want to fool around," I told him. "I want to see what these enzymes can do."

This time, I had patients take them between meals. That way, with no digestion going on, the protease enzymes would make it through the stomach and into the intestines, where they could be absorbed and sent wherever the body needed them.

It became very evident immediately how these enzymes were going to be useful. Consistently among my patients, I was finding areas in the body where there seemed to be diminished bone pain.

There are very specific areas of the body under physical stress because of gravity. Structural stress. I'm referring to the weight-bearing parts of the legs—the shins, in particular. This is the area where my athlete patients were having their pain. Their legs were stressed from running on concrete or asphalt. And that's where the pain was relieved in particular—patients with shin splints were having less pain.

So I had Tony double the dose, the concentration. This time around, I noticed from my urinalysis tests that my patients were becoming slightly calcium deficient. Meanwhile, more protease meant more complete digestion of protein, and bone is made up of protein. So what I was seeing in these 30 patients told me that protease enzymes would relieve shin pain.

I finally had something I could count on consistently.

What I didn't get at this point was that the protease was also making the immune system stronger.

I was about to experience this first-hand, when I started taking the blend myself.

A Shot In The Dark

What was the reason I started taking the protease supplements myself? Because I wanted to boost the dose even higher, and I needed to see what (if any) problems the dosage might cause before I started giving larger doses to my patients.

It was all about patient safety.

And yet, in the back of my mind I was also thinking about what I had read in Dr. Howell's book about leukocytosis, about the digestive demands being placed on the immune system.

Even more to the point, there was an article in *Scientific American*

Chapter 1—Desire

I'd read back in 1967 and never forgotten. The article described how disease-fighting white blood cells kill bacteria and viruses by injecting them with protease enzymes. Inside each white blood cell is a lysosome package containing protease enzymes. Illustrations in the article showed how a white blood cell gets belly to belly with a bacteria, and how it uses calcium as a trigger to literally shoot the protease into the bacteria, which would then be destroyed.

So here I was getting protease enzymes across the intestinal walls and into the bloodstream by giving the enzymes between meals. They were going systemic, to wherever the body needed them.

Once again I asked Collier to double the dose—raise the activity level—of the protease supplement I had been giving to my patients. Again, I was looking to test safety.

He did so, and I took the capsules.

Two or three days passed. Nothing happened.

"Double it again," I said.

"Okay, but be careful," Collier said. He hadn't made anything that strong before.

So I took the capsules again. This time I had a rip-roaring pain in my ears like no pain I had felt since my tonsils were taken out.

My ears felt literally on fire with inflammation.

The first thing I thought? I should go to the emergency room. But this was by no means the first time I had been through that pain.

I sat down to think about what was going on. I had an active bacteria, and my body had never attacked it. Now for the very first time, at this third dosage of protease enzymes, my fully armed immune cells were on the attack. But it wasn't enough to kill the bacteria. I had started a brawl, and I couldn't finish it.

I needed more enzymes!

So I went to Collier. "Look," I said. "We've attacked this infection in my ears, but we're not strong enough to win. You have to double this one more time."

That's when he really balked. But I said, "You have to do this. I know you can do it."

He did increase the dose, and I took some calcium with it, because I had already found the protease supplement caused calcium deficiencies in high doses.

Eureka! It stopped it cold. Within 36 hours, the infection was gone. And it has *never* come back.

I had lived with this infection for 43 years—from 1938 to 1980—and I had finally won the battle.

I've been up to my ears in enzymes ever since.

Food *for* Thought

It is not my intention to turn this book into a personal memoir, but rather to take you along a learning curve that has opened my eyes and changed my life as a health care provider.

CHAPTER 2

PREPARATION

It's one thing to have an epiphany; it's quite another to put it to work for you.

Ending the 43-year-long infection in my ears, thanks to my double-double dose of protease, was just such an epiphany. And yet, while I was able to wear an inside-the-ear hearing aid for the first time in my life, I was still no better off in my understanding of how to use digestive enzymes and other dietary supplements to relieve my patients' visceral symptoms. These symptoms originate not from structural issues, but rather from internal, organic stress. That understanding would come to me over the next five years.

The past 12 years, leading up to my 1980 epiphany, had by no means been wasted.

For one thing, I had learned my craft and the key principles that infused my work with value as both a science and as a healing art.

> **If there is one element unique to the chiropractic field, it is that the structural and visceral aspects of the human body are inextricably connected and must be perceived and treated as such.**

The development of this integrated human system begins during the third week (16th day) of human embryonic development—when the nervous system, internal organs, and musculoskeletal system grow out of three distinct "germ layers." These leaf-like embryonic layers were first observed by the German physiologist Caspar Friedrich Wolff in 1759.

The outer layer, or ectoderm, evolves to become the skin, the hair, the nails, the upper respiratory tract, and the brain and spinal cord. The middle layer, or mesoderm, becomes the musculoskeletal system, the body's connective tissues, the circulatory system and the lymphatic system. The innermost layer, or endoderm, forms the body's working organs.

While all this is taking place, the spinal cord is busy sending out nerve fibers, connecting these three layers to receptors in the skin, the muscles, and all the organs of the body. It is through this hard-wired "neuro-switchboard" that the brain will receive and send messages, regulating all body functions in times of normalcy and in times of stress.

Now consider that messages, or impulses, relayed through this switchboard travel along a *party line*. In other words, when an organ

Chapter 2—Preparation

is struggling and sends a distress signal to the brain, the returning message goes out on the party line to other organs of the body as well. In the case of a struggling gall bladder, this can result in involuntary muscle contraction around the shoulder.

Thus, as a chiropractor, I learned that pain in a patient's shoulder may have nothing to do with a structural injury to that shoulder. The pain may be visceral—the outward expression of a stressed gallbladder or other organ having trouble doing its job. And all the adjustment in the world will not make this pain go away permanently. It will be back with the next meal.

Two prominent researchers whose early work gave rise to this understanding were Henry Head and James MacKenzie.

Sir Henry Head was one of the principal developers of clinical neuroscience. Among his many accomplishments was the mapping out of human dermatomes—areas of the skin served by sensory neurons rooted in the spinal cord. Studying patients suffering from shingles, Head was able to trace their surface pain directly to its corresponding roots in their spinal nerves, with the specific area of the skin experiencing the pain corresponding to a specific section of the spinal cord.

This work was published in 1900.

Furthermore, Head found, diseases involving the internal organs can produce these same surface symptoms and other "tender areas" of visceral disease when impulses from the brain are sent out along the party line.

Anytime an organ is under stress and not functioning properly, measurable changes will occur on the skin, according to Head. That's what his mapping out of human dermatomes revealed. Then there was Sir James Mackenzie, a Scottish cardiologist known for his pioneering work in cardiac arrhythmias. Mackenzie noted in 1917 that there are two kinds of muscle contractions in the human body—voluntary and involuntary. Voluntary muscle contractions are associated with specific body functions (e.g., the scratching of one's nose); involuntary muscle contractions (e.g., the twitching of an eye), he called "viscera-motor reflexes."

Unlike voluntary contractions, MacKenzie found that involuntary contractions do not necessarily result in a shortening of the muscle. Nor do they necessarily involve the entire length of the muscle. Further, an involuntary muscle contraction is not subject to fatigue, so it can last for an indefinite time. And so the struggling gallbladder can produce chronic shoulder pain.

The finely tuned chiropractor can distinguish between a structural or visceral cause of involuntary muscle contractions.

What I found during the first few months of my practice was that most of the musculoskeletal complaints coming my way were, in fact, visceral in origin. An organ—the stomach, gallbladder, pancreas, prostate, uterus, breast, whatever—was not doing what it was supposed to do, because the organ was under stress. That stress was causing an involuntary muscle contraction, which caused loss of range of motion in the joint.

There is a much larger picture emerging from these observations. It has to do with the concept of *universal intelligence* as it applies to the science-based healing art of chiropractic, and other healing arts going back to the ancients.

We will see more about universal intelligence later in this chapter.

It's all about maintaining homeostasis. And this is where chiropractic really captured my imagination.

Universal Intelligence

Taken broadly, universal intelligence has been described as "the intrinsic tendency for things to self-organize and co-evolve into ever more complex, intricately interwoven and mutually compatible forms."

On a more personal note, one might say that each of us is a universe unto ourselves, with every cellular aspect of our life functions orchestrated by the same universal intelligence that has done so in all living creatures since the beginning of time.

D.D. Palmer had such a vision when he adopted the term as the founding principle for his chiropractic philosophy. "As the Intelligent Energy that operates the human machine is derived from an Infinite Source," he wrote, "it is limited only by the capacity of the brain to transform and individualize it." Further, "Any excess, deficiency, or irregularity of action, either of which is a form of disease, must be due to some mechanical obstruction which prevents its normal transmission." We think again of the switchboard and all its components. This image illustrates the universal intelligence that enables all our body cells and organ systems to function as intended, in homeostatic harmony.

What Is Homeostasis?

The word *homeostasis*, as it applies here, was coined by the American physiologist Walter B. Cannon in 1930 from the Greek words "same" and "steady" to describe how the human body maintains an *internal environment* conducive to the healthy functioning of all of its cells.

Certain fundamental activities are common to almost all cells and represent the minimal requirements for maintaining cell integrity and life.

These activities include:

- Taking food from the surrounding environment and excreting waste back into that environment
- Producing energy by breaking down these organic nutrients and making new molecules from them
- Reproducing themselves
- Consistently demonstrating the desire to live.

In this sense, every cell in the human body shares these same fundamental requirements with the single-cell amoeba. But, because of their specialized functions, human cells require that their oxygen and nutrients be delivered to them, and their wastes removed for them. It is the extracellular fluid in which all body cells live and breathe, so to speak, which acts as a nutritional delivery and waste removal system.

Let's take a look at this internal environment.

Sixty percent of the total human body weight is water. The fluid inside the cells (intracellular fluid) accounts for two-thirds of the total body water. The fluid outside the cells (extracellular fluid) accounts for the other third. It is only the extracellular fluid bathing the cells that must remain relatively constant in terms of acid-alkaline balance (pH), temperature, volume (the amount of water), and levels of dissolved substances needed to nourish the cells, such as sugar, protein, cholesterol and iron.

That is homeostasis. And it must be maintained if cells and organ systems are to function in a healthy manner.

While microscopic studies have identified about 200 different types of cells in the human body, all human cells are derived from four broad categories of cells based on the functions they perform. These are: muscle cells, nerve cells, epithelial cells, and connective tissue cells.

Finally, there are the body's 10 organ systems, all of which contribute to maintaining homeostasis of the body systems within the internal environment:

Circulatory	Musculoskeletal
Digestive	Nervous
Endocrine	Reproductive
Immune	Respiratory
Integumentary (skin)	Urinary

These 10 organ systems exist for one reason only—to provide an internal environment and act as a life-support system for all of the body's individual cells. In the vernacular, somebody's got to grow the food; somebody's got to build the houses; somebody's got to supply the electricity; somebody's got to stand guard; somebody's got to deliver the groceries; somebody's got to pick up the garbage; somebody's got to create energy; and so on.

The body has two major control systems for maintaining homeostasis.

The autonomic, or involuntary nervous system, functions below our conscious thoughts to control functions like heart rate, digestion, respiratory rate, salivation, perspiration, sexual arousal, and so on.

Then there's the endocrine system—the glands that secrete hormones. These include the pituitary gland; the pancreas, which also secretes digestive enzymes outside the body into the digestive tract; the ovaries; the thyroid gland; the testes; and the adrenal glands.

Both of these systems receive signals and direction from the brain—more specifically, from the hypothalamus, which is seated just above the brain stem.

While the hypothalamus is not exposed directly to the extracellular fluid, it does control and regulate the temperature, volume and concentration of everything in the extracellular fluids.

The hypothalamus has been called the "Master" endocrine gland, because it regulates the entire endocrine system, and more.

When it comes to maintaining homeostasis, with regard to oversight and management, the hypothalamus pretty much runs the show. But when it comes to troops on the ground, protein is king.

About Protein

There are two kinds of protein in the body. There's protein that cells use for growth and repair, which can also be converted to energy. And then there are the blood-borne plasma proteins, which maintain homeostasis. Plasma proteins transport nutrients; they detoxify waste; they maintain pH by buffering excess acidity or alkalinity; and they maintain the fluid balance in the extracellular fluid.

It's protein that maintains calcium in the blood. At any given time, roughly 50 percent of the calcium in the blood will be free-floating, while 50 percent will be bound to protein. This ratio will never change.

A protein deficiency will rarely show up in a blood test, because protein is essential in maintaining homeostasis, and the brain will pull protein into the blood from wherever it must. Protein deficiency often only shows up in a blood test in the late stages of disease. Calcium showing up in the urine, however, *is* a sign of protein deficiency, because the brain will dump calcium to maintain the 50/50 ratio between free-floating calcium and calcium bound to protein.

Maintaining homeostasis in the body's intracellular fluids is the number one priority for the universal intelligence that is born into each and every one of us. Any deviation produces stress and, eventually, disease.

And so the orchestration continues.

Just look at how the body makes stomach acid. It's absolutely mind-boggling.

Stomach acid, or hydrochloric acid (HCl), doesn't exist in the body between meals. It's the stretching of the stomach when it receives food that signals the brain to make hydrochloric acid, and this process takes at least 45 minutes.

HCl production starts when carbon dioxide leaves the bloodstream and enters the parietal cells in the lining of the stomach, where the enzyme carbonic anhydrase causes it to combine with water to form carbonic acid.

The carbonic acid is then broken down into bicarbonate ions and hydrogen ions.

The bicarbonate ions are transported back into the blood, and the hydrogen is transported into the stomach.

In the meantime, chloride and potassium in the blood are being exchanged for sodium. The chloride then combines with the hydrogen in the stomach to form hydrochloric acid, which will then be used to convert pepsinogen into protein-digesting pepsin.

Hydrochloric acid does not itself digest protein, or anything else for that matter.

The tricky part in all this is maintaining the right pH level in the blood.

Taking carbon dioxide, which is acid, out of the blood, and returning bicarbonate, which is alkaline pushes the blood in an alkaline direction. If the blood becomes too alkaline, the body winds up in the emergency room in metabolic alkalosis. The necessary magic is performed by dropping alkalinity out of the blood through the kidney.

That's why every time we eat, our urine becomes alkaline.

It's all about maintaining homeostasis, or paying the price.

Hydrochloric acid also keeps the bile thin so it can degrease the fat we consume and allow our digestive enzymes to penetrate it. When we are HCl deficient, the bile in the body becomes thick and doesn't flow adequately. The biliary system becomes stressed—whether you still have your gallbladder or not—and we wind up with gas and bloating, constipation, headaches, and, yes, shoulder pain

And so, the wheel comes full circle.

When it comes to maintaining homeostasis, stress is the enemy.

That's the key in all of this.

Learning About Stress

It was in the late 1960s, right at the time of my chiropractic training, that Hans Selye's book, *The Stress of Life*, to be followed by *Stress Without Distress*, were bringing his life's work on stress to world attention. That work, documented over four decades by 1,700 research papers, along with seven popular books, had earned Selye

Chapter 2—Preparation

eight Nobel Prize nominations and the acclaim of all those in the healing arts.

He taught the world about stress.

Selye proved that stress is not a vague or undefinable term having only to do with our being unloved, overworked and underpaid. Rather, he showed that the human body responds to any kind of stress, be it mechanical, chemical or emotional, in a very specific and predictable way.

Selye called this response by the body the "general adaptation syndrome."

It starts with the body in a state of health, or normalcy. If a "stimulus stress" is applied that requires a change to maintain normalcy, a signal is sent to the brain, which in turn sends out signals producing a resistance reaction. If the stimulus disappears and was not strong enough to cause tissue damage, then we probably don't even notice the reaction that has taken place.

Many such reactions occur every day as we adjust our rates of respiration and heartbeat, as well as countless hormonal and autonomic nerve responses, to meet changes and challenges in our environment—both external and internal.

If the stimulus continues, those parts of the body affected must elicit aid from other tissues, or use more and more nutrients to maintain their heightened state of function. This situation will continue without issue, as long as the flow of nutrition is maintained and the waste products produced by the affected organ/tissue are transported away and are not allowed to accumulate.

However, once tissues under stress become fatigued because of a lack of continuing support from related tissues or organs, nutrition, or waste removal, or because the stimulus is simply too strong, we enter a state of exhaustion.

It is at this point that we begin to experience symptoms. The area of stress has become a sort of demilitarized zone, a no-man's-land. Affected tissues are not exhausted to the point of damage. Objective findings, from physical examination (except for palpation of involuntary muscle contractions and alterations on a 24-hour urine sample), blood tests, and X-rays, are all still negative. We have not yet entered the zone of disease. And yet, health has not been maintained.

The big question now is, which way do we move next? Up to health? Or down to disease, degeneration, and eventually death?

Now here's the key.

Selye's findings demonstrate that since the human body has its own specific ways of maintaining normal function, and therefore health, any healing attempts should be directed at relieving the stress and providing nutrients for the body to use in its own defense—and its own healing process.

Such efforts, in conjunction with removing excessive waste that always results when cells are stressed and stimulated, would unquestionably fall within the province of nutrition.

For Selye, the best way to help a body under stress is to provide the right nutrition to restore homeostasis and normal function to the stressed system or systems, before the body reaches a state of disease.

Unfortunately, Selye's work has not been fully appreciated and applied as often and judiciously as it should be. The preference has been more in favor of finding drugs (both prescription or over-the-counter) to cover up symptoms, or early warning signs of stress. And stress long camouflaged and ignored leads most often to disease, not health and well-being.

Of course, it should be obvious that a patient with disease—just like a patient without disease—requires good nutrition, as well as

Chapter 2—Preparation

dietary supplementation to meet the increased demands being placed on the body.

All of this was very much in keeping with my chiropractic training—to recognize the human body's need to maintain homeostasis, and to determine and provide whatever was needed to deal with the stress at hand, be it emotional, mechanical or chemical in nature, *and* before the symptoms that had brought that patient to my office reached a state of disease.

I had my tools ready.

First was the taking of the patient's history. What kind of emotional stress were they going through that might produce a weakness in the body? What injuries or surgeries had they had in the past? What medications were they taking that might produce the symptoms that had brought them to my office, or be camouflaging the underlying problem?

Then came the physical exam—listening to the heart and the lungs; looking at the patient's posture, including things like head tilt, whether the shoulders and hips are level; looking at knee flex and ankle pronation; looking for involuntary muscle contraction.

Muscle contraction at the base of the skull may be found on either side of head tilt. A low hip is indicative of weakness in the pelvis and legs. Knee flexion usually occurs on the side of the long leg and may lead to future hip replacement. With ankle pronation, both arches falling evenly are not as much of a problem as when one arch falls more than the other. If left uncorrected, there is continual stress to the body with every step the patient takes.

Looking for muscle contraction, we try and figure out *why* the muscle is contracted and where it's coming from. Are we fighting against gravity, or is the contraction coming from a struggling organ?

It was a constant learning process from the day I started my practice.

When a patient comes in with right knee problems, chiropractic students are taught to look at not only the knee, but the ankle or the pelvis as well. So I treated this particular patient's ankle and hip, and she didn't get better. The problem, it turned out, was actually in the other leg. The one she complained about was simply working too hard. So I treated her other leg, and suddenly the pain went away on the other side.

It was the most amazing thing.

The visceral problems were the most vexing.

My Awakening

As mentioned earlier, within the first three months of starting my practice, I found that most of my patients were not coming to me with musculoskeletal problems. They had musculoskeletal complaints, but the cause of the structural problem was not rooted in structure. It was of visceral origin. Some organ was under stress and not doing its job, resulting in muscle contraction.

Again, the chiropractor can adjust the joint and relieve the pain, but the next time he sees the patient, it's back. And he can't figure out why.

It's what I've come to call the second factor in chiropractic.

The question was, how to get to the source of the problem? In a perfect world, this information would have been at my fingertips, but it was not.

Chapter 2—Preparation

I had studied the concept of homeostasis in college. It was a pretty straightforward explanation of how the body maintains equilibrium in the fluids that surround its various systems and organs. But it would be another 12 years before I would finally accumulate the knowledge on my own to really address the visceral aspect of my patients' symptoms.

The tools to do so, however, were there from the beginning. We had very dependable blood and urine tests. It was just a matter of learning how to use them, and what to do once I knew what was going on.

The 24-hour urinalysis, for example, where we collect urine from the patient over a 24-hour period, consists of nine tests that have been around for over 100 years. The body is supposed to put out a certain amount of calcium, so if it's not showing up in the urine, you know the body is calcium deficient. If it's eliminating more calcium than it should, that may mean it doesn't have enough protein to hold onto it. So the patient has a protein deficiency. This is how I figured out that the patients I was giving protease enzymes to in Chapter 1 were becoming calcium deficient—because there wasn't any calcium showing up in their 24-hour urine tests.

Then there's the blood test that's used to measure inflammation. You draw blood, add an anticoagulant to prevent it from clotting, and leave it sit in a tube for 24 hours. During that time, the red blood cells separate from the serum and fall to the bottom. The faster they fall, the more inflamed the patient is.

But there's more. It's the way these red blood cells stack up—or don't—as they settle at the bottom of the tube, that is more telling. When there is disease in the body, they clump together in two different patterns. When they clump one on top of the other, it is called Rouleaux. This can occur when there is acute tissue damage, or simply because the patient is too alkaline.

When the red blood cells clump together like iron filings at the end of a magnet, it's a sign that the blood is being stressed in an acid direction. It wouldn't be until I learned how to use food enzymes that I could make changes to these stress-induced results.

So urine and blood tests can be used to detect various deficiencies.

The question in my mind was, how do you correct such a deficiency?

I recall one day at Logan College. I was taking classes in structure. I had just come from X-ray class looking at spines, and I was all excited, telling a buddy as we were walking towards the cafeteria that this is what I was going to do with the rest of my life.

He said, "That's very nice, Howard, what are you going to do with somebody who's anemic? What bone are you going to adjust? How are you going to get iron into that patient? Put a rusty nail in your hand and drive it into him that way?"

We both laughed. Then I thought about it. What structural problems would you see in a patient with an iron deficiency? Does iron deficiency produce a specific structural problem that you can recognize without doing blood work? And how would you deliver the iron?

That's where it all started for me. When I got into practice and could see the magnitude of the visceral aspect, I knew I had to figure it out.

I spent the next years, more than a decade, trying to correlate vitamins and mineral supplements, along with digestive enzyme supplements, looking for any consistent benefit in relieving patient symptoms.

I tried everything. I used all the vitamins, all the minerals. I used all the protomorphogens—ground-up tissues from various sources. You can buy protomorphogens for any organ in the body—ground-up bone, ground-up pancreas, ground-up duodenum, heart, liver,

Chapter 2—Preparation

spleen—all with the theory of supplementing a specific protein from a specific organ, basically anything the patient may be deficient in.

But it didn't work consistently.

I tried free-form amino acids. Back in the 70s, the world was going to be saved by isolating individual amino acids. The problem is, the human body is very selective about its amino acids. It's like a symphony orchestra, where the brain is the conductor and it wants 27 violins, seven cellos, a certain mix of horns, and only one cymbalist. And, no matter what happens, it is not going to change that relationship—that ratio. So if you're taking an amino acid supplement that will disturb that ratio, the body will not absorb it. It all comes back to universal intelligence and maintaining homeostasis.

So they didn't work either. There was no consistent benefit I could count on.

What I found during those 12 years was that supplements simply don't work, unless you happen to touch on a particular deficiency. So when Tony Collier came to me and asked me to formulate products, I told him that would be easy. Just tell me what the symptoms are of a protease, amylase, lipase or cellulase deficiency, and I can do it. But he couldn't tell me. Remember? No one knew the answer, not even old Doc Howell.

> **After the 100 patients I treated with protease enzymes, and after treating my own ears, I was still pretty much in the dark. What was I supposed to do, wait for somebody to come in with shin splints or an ear infection? I had to have more than that. I knew I couldn't be practicing on symptoms alone.**

And so I was back to universal intelligence. What I was looking for was the common denominator. With all this, with all these vitamin and mineral supplements, with the body trying to maintain homeostasis, what is needed? What is the common denominator that I can work with as a healer? It definitely wasn't in my education yet. And nobody else had the answer. But somebody had to have it.

How does one go about getting a functional "handle" on universal intelligence? Perhaps by going back to the beginning? It seemed like a good idea. So I turned to the ancient healing arts, in search of that common denominator.

The Search

I began with the ancient healing system of Ayurveda, which originated more than 3,000 years ago in India and exists today as one of that country's traditional health care systems.

Like other ancient healing systems, Ayurveda subscribed to the concept of opposites—for every living thing or situation there is an exact opposite and the two exist in a state of tension with each other.

Hence, we have white and black, male and female, positive and negative, material and spiritual, left and right, outer and inner, heavier and lighter, and so on.

In physiological terms, there was acute and chronic, parasympathetic and sympathetic, circulation of blood/lymph and generation of blood and lymph, and so forth.

In terms of diagnostics, there was hot and cold, dry and wet, external and internal.

Chapter 2—Preparation

Life was an endless fluctuation between opposites—from the ancients right up to today's practitioners of Western medicine.

Ayurveda

The Hindis built Ayurveda around three humors, or Doshas—Kapha, Pitta and Vata. The impulse principle, Vata, mobilizes the functioning of the nervous system. Vata is composed of air and space, and is therefore characterized as light, petite, cool and dry. Pitta is the energy principle, which uses bile to direct digestion and metabolism into the venous system. Pitta is composed of fire and water, and is hot and acid. Kapha is the body fluid principle, which relates to mucous, lubrication and the carrier of nutrients into the arterial system. It is composed of water and earth, and is large, heavy, cold and wet.

Could this correlation of three, I wondered, connect with the three embryologic layers—the ectoderm, the mesoderm and the endoderm? Not exactly. I was just trying to find a common thread to Western medicine through the cultural bias of this ancient healing system.

However, the balance of these three bodily humors equals health, and imbalance equals ill health. So we're back to homeostasis.

Treatment of imbalances by Ayurvedic practitioners consists of herbs—hundreds of them—as well as various animal products and minerals.

I couldn't make any sense of the minerals. I couldn't compare it to my Western education.

I did find some things interesting, though. I was also fascinated by their classification of herbs and how to use them and when. From my Western perspective, I understood the pharmaceutical concept of isolating the "active ingredient" from an herb and concentrating it. In my experience, using whole herbs would be hit-or-miss depending on the ability or inability of the patient to digest the herb. And yet, the Ayurvedic doctor was concentrating the right nutrients into the patient, using whole food sources, and controlling the diet—something I couldn't do with most of my patients.

So I turned to Chinese medicine, still searching for my common denominator.

Traditional Chinese Medicine

Chinese medicine was first introduced in this country when *New York Times* journalist, James "Scotty" Reston, accompanying President Nixon's Secretary of State Henry Kissinger on a trip to China, required an emergency appendectomy. Acupuncture was used as the only anesthesia. Besides making national news, the procedure was so effective that doctors from the UCLA pain clinic made subsequent visits to China, and brought acupuncture back to the United States to be used alongside conventional therapies.

Traditional Chinese medicine was founded on the principle that the human body is a miniature version of the all-encompassing universe. The two opposing but complementary forces of yin and yang support health, and disease occurs when these forces are out of balance.

Again, we're into opposites.

Chinese medicine is practiced on 12 meridians, and the flow of energy through these meridians, or energy pathways, each involves a different organ system. The liver meridian starts at the big toe and runs up into the face. It's named for the liver simply because it runs through the liver. If the liver is struggling, there will be a flow of energy along that pathway. This disrupted flow of energy from the struggling organ can result in—you guessed it—an involuntary muscle contraction.

Acupuncture is an effort to balance the flow of energy in the body by inserting pins along these meridians. University of Vermont researchers using ultrasound imaging recently mapped out a correlation between traditional acupuncture points and connective tissue layers, suggesting that meridians are in fact located in connective tissue. Anything that affects the connective tissue, which holds the body together and supports everything, will affect posture. And any resulting muscle contractions can be traced back to the organ under stress.

Meanwhile, I was still looking for that common denominator.

Traditional Chinese medicine envisioned five elements–fire, earth, wood, metal, and water—representing the stages of human life, the functioning of the body, and its fluctuations with disease. More specifically, the five elements corresponded to different organ systems. Fire corresponded to the small intestine and the heart; earth corresponded to the stomach and the spleen; wood corresponded to the gallbladder and the liver; metal corresponded to the large intestine and the lungs; and water corresponded to the bladder and the kidney.

Moreover, each was associated with elements like human emotion, the turn of the season, taste, color, sound. It was all about the universal order of all things in the world and in ourselves.

So how did these five elements apply to my search for the common denominator? This unfortunately was not within my Western grasp. That is, I couldn't connect it to my Western thinking.

So I turned to the third ancient healing system, the Greek-Persian tradition of Unani-Tibb, which originated from the teachings of the ancient Greek physicians Hippocrates and Galen and gave rise to Western medicine.

And this is where the magic happened for me.

The Magic Number

The magic number in Unani-Tibb is four. The human body is made up of four elements: Earth, Air, Water and Fire. Each has its own temperament—hot, cold, wet and dry.

Again, we're into opposites.

Further, the Unani-Tibb system is built around four body humors: Blood, Phlegm, Yellow Bile and Black Bile. The unique mixture of these substances in an individual determines that person's temperament. A predominance of Blood humor gives a person a sanguine temperament (cheerfully optimistic); a dominance of Phlegm humor renders that person phlegmatic (calm); Yellow Bile makes one bilious (bad tempered, spiteful, irritable); and a person with an abundance of Black Bile humor is overcome by melancholy (pensively sad, gloomy, depressed).

These humors have been ascribed to legendary literary characters. Both Sophocles's *Oedipus* and Shakespeare's *Hamlet* have been described as melancholic, owing to an accumulation of Black Bile.

Furthermore, each humor has its own temperament. Blood is hot and moist; Phlegm is cold and moist; Yellow Bile is hot and dry; and Black Bile is cold and dry.

Hippocrates was known to have his patients lie down in muddy water, after which he would look for areas on their bodies where the mud had dried up, revealing *hot spots*.

When the four humors and the four temperaments (hot, cold, dry, moist) are all in *equilibrium*, the person is in good health. When the equilibrium is disturbed, body functions become abnormal and the person is in a state of disease. Once again, we're back to homeostasis.

Of particular interest to me was the fact that when a person becomes a Unani-Tibb practitioner, he or she specializes in one of the four stages of digestion:

- Gastric digestion
- Hepatic (liver) digestion
- Vessel digestion, in which every tissue derives its nutrition
- Tissue digestion, which converts nutritional elements into tissue, with the waste materials remaining in the humors excreted.

This is the point I had my "Aha! moment."

It just hit me one night. It was all about digestion. What the Ayurvedic practitioners were looking at was whether an herb produced *heat* when you digested it. That's what the Greeks were looking at too: Does it produce heat?

And that's what the Chinese were looking at: Is this fire?

Or is it cold? Black Bile is cold.

What all these systems were looking at was creating acidity or alkalinity, or bringing water to or drying out the human body. That's what all the ancients were doing, and I could do it with food and enzymes—food for nutritional value to correct deficiencies, and enzymes to predigest the food and deliver it across an incompetent digestive system, rendered so by our modern day, enzyme-deficient diet.

It was all Western chemistry.

Nutrients associated with acidity include sulfur, phosphorous and chloride. Those associated with alkalinity include sodium, potassium and magnesium. Acidity, in turn, is associated with heat, and alkalinity is associated with cold.

Where do acid nutrients come from? Meat, cheese and eggs. Where do alkaline nutrients come from? Vegetables and fruit.

It was all coming together.

What creates heat? Protein. If someone tends to have cold hands, they are protein deficient. If someone gets red in the face when they laugh, and they have an abundance of energy and can party forever, never get tired, and go right to work early the next morning, they are high in protein. Protein is what athletes eat before they hit the athletic field. High-protein foods drive people, and they drive emotions.

The ancients knew this. But they didn't have concentrated enzymes to work with, to deliver what was needed to correct deficiencies. But I did.

The other part of the four-element system in Unani-Tibb was wet and dry. Those are the vitamins. Vitamins are either water soluble or fat soluble. Now all of a sudden, I could mix the minerals and vitamins and food and the enzymes—and put it all together.

I could do the same thing Hippocrates had done. It's just that he had everything in his food supply in ancient Greece, including the enzymes. Nowadays, the food enzymes have been cooked and processed, and genetically engineered out of everything we eat. So I had to put the enzymes back, using supplements.

Suddenly I could figure out what my patients were deficient in and give it to them.

I could see it in their urinalysis and in a complete blood count.

Whatever the body has too much of, it throws into the urine, and whatever it doesn't have enough of, it holds onto. Moreover, the 24-hour urinalysis, in terms of overall volume and the amount of chloride in the blood, matched up with Hippocrates's four humors.

People with high overall volume of urine during the 24-hour period and high chloride content are burning protein as their chief source of energy. They fall into Hippocrates's hot and moist Blood humor category.

Those with high urine volume and low chloride content rely on simple carbohydrates as their chief source of fuel and belong to the Phlegm humor.

Those with low overall volume and high chloride during the 24-hour collection period burn fats as their chief source of energy. They are Yellow Bile.

And those with low overall volume and low chlorides use complex carbohydrates as their chief fuel. They are full of Black Bile if they struggle to digest them.

You can see the same thing in a complete blood count.

In Buffy Coat Analysis, blood is drawn, put in a centrifuge and spun until it separates into four layers. Those layers also correspond to the Greek humors.

The top frothy, transparent layer is the blood platelets. This corresponds to the Phlegm humor.

The second layer down, which is yellowish-green, consists of the white blood cells. This corresponds to the Bile humor.

The next layer down, which is clear red, is hematocrit, and corresponds to the Blood humor.

And the fourth layer down, which is made up of red blood cells, is thick and black and corresponds to Black Bile.

What can be said about a person with Phlegm humor? These people eat too much sugar, because they don't digest fat. They are depleting alkaline minerals, particularly potassium and magnesium, and sodium. Magnesium, while it has many applications, is used especially in protein metabolism. The most outstanding symptoms among people with magnesium deficiencies are emotional imbalances. People who are potassium deficient have stiff, sore joints, or hypoflexia. And they are constipated. They have heart arrhythmias and difficulty processing thought. It's in the medical literature. They are very *phlegmatic.*

The Bile person is struggling with bile production. As a result, they have difficulty digesting fat and protein. They tend to be argumentative. They are not positive. The glass is always half empty. They are very frustrated and can be very angry and feverish.

The Blood person gets energy from protein. They function very well on all levels. They can process thought; they are more athletic; they are good speakers and good thinkers. Protein, remember, maintains homeostasis. And they have good liver function and good bile. But they must maintain good digestion.

The Black Bile person is melancholy. They are toxic because they are not digesting well and they're not eliminating well. They lack energy. *I can't seem to get through the day,* they complain. *I'm just so sad and ... melancholy.* I came to learn that this mental state can be brought on by the inability to digest adequately, regardless of the type of diet.

The ancients, I found during my investigations, all looked at the same basic picture—the body's struggle to maintain homeostasis—with diet playing a major role in an individual's health.

It all connects up.

> **But the key, the common denominator I was looking for—the missing link—was the digestive enzymes needed to deliver the right nutrition to the struggling organ system.**
> **In a word, the Workers.**

The fact is, neither vitamins nor minerals or any of the other nutritional elements our body cells need to function are workers.

They do no actual work. It's the enzymes that do the work. They are the workers. Without them, there is nothing. So let's move on.

Food *for* Thought

Over the next five years, I would learn how to know what was needed and how to use Nature's workers to deliver the necessary nutrition past an incompetent digestive system to restore homeostasis and relieve my patients' visceral symptoms.

Chapter 3

Action

So enzymes were the key.

Not pancreatic enzyme supplements, which do not predigest foods, and which I had tried without success, but Howell's food enzymes, which do their predigestive work in the "food enzyme stomach."

They were the means by which I would be able to move needed nutrition to struggling organs and past an incompetent digestive system.

If only life were that simple.

The question now became how to deliver what to where—i.e., what specific nutrition each organ system needed, and what specific food enzyme was needed to make that delivery.

Oh yes, and how to determine which organ system was under stress and in need of nutrition.

The Enzyme Advantage

That learning process would take place over the next five years.

Once again, I sat in my living room contemplating yet another square one.

My investigations into the ancient healing arts had taught me that they were all involved with the concept of opposites—i.e., hot and cold, wet and dry, etc. They were all looking at deviations from normal. They knew nothing about physiology or biochemistry. The word homeostasis didn't even exist for them.

So there I was with my Western education, trying to figure out how I was going to translate and apply that principle, and perhaps teach it to other health care providers someday. That thought had entered my mind. I couldn't very well go out teaching enzymes through an acupuncture or Ayurvedic window. That wasn't going to cut it for a Western audience. Or me, for that matter.

It was all about maintaining homeostasis. That was the Holy Grail of the physical body, according to modern Western physiology.

> **Everybody in Western medicine knows what homeostasis is. But nobody pays attention to it. The Western approach is to simply treat symptoms. What was the key to diagnosing and treating the underlying cause, before full-blown disease has a chance to develop?**

That was Western enough. I just needed a way in.

I thought about it, and then it hit me.

Chapter 3—Action

It's All About Energy

Homeostasis doesn't just happen; it doesn't come automatically. The body is in a constant, 24/7, 365-day-a-year struggle to do this. It follows that every organ system, every tissue in the body, must have adequate nutrition to perform its role in maintaining homeostasis within the extracellular fluids—despite ever-changing challenges.

And this ongoing organic process doesn't happen without a cost.

Looking at it another way, we're all being taxed for this service, which involves the delivery of nutrition and the pickup of waste from all our body cells.

The question now became, how do we pay for that service? The answer was right there in plain sight. It's *energy*.

It's all about energy—the ebb and flow of energy within each of the 10 organ systems as they perform their part in maintaining homeostasis.

And enzymes—Nature's workers—were at the very heart of it.

Once again, I was on my way.

As I mentioned earlier, it was Dr. Edward Howell who opened the door to enzymes for me. It was his life's work.

Howell shared his two seminal books, *Enzyme Nutrition* and *Food Enzymes for Health and Longevity*, with me when I visited with him at his retirement home in Ft. Myers, Florida, on several occasions in 1982. Those visits changed my attitude about nutrition. I learned about the importance of food enzymes—the "missing link" in human nutrition.

The son of German immigrants, Howell graduated from the University of Illinois Medical School in 1924. His first job was at the Lindlahr Sanitarium in Elmhurst, just outside of Chicago. The Lindlahr was a naturopathic mecca for more than 80,000 patients worldwide. It was the Mayo Clinic of its time, treating chronic degenerative diseases with a combination of fasting and fruit juices to purge the body of poisons and give it time to heal. The Lindlahr offered patients raw food diets, hydrotherapy, osteopathy, chiropractic, massage, various herbal remedies, and plenty of exercise and plenty of rest.

The turning point for Doc Howell came in 1928, when two Lindlahr staples—daily doses of freshly squeezed orange juice and fresh butter applied to patients' skin—stopped producing therapeutic benefits. Suddenly, patients' gastrointestinal problems and skin conditions (eczema, psoriasis, etc.), were back with a vengeance.

It made no sense, until one of the nurses told Howell that the butter was no longer coming from the local dairy, and the orange juice was no longer being fresh squeezed in the kitchen. Both items were now arriving by truck from distributors—pasteurized.

Nobody at the Lindlahr had even heard the term pasteurization.

Howell met with scientists from the canning industry to find out what pasteurization involved. He learned that it was all about using heat to kill off what they called the "life element" in these products, in order to increase shelf life. They did kill off bacteria, yes, so disease would not breed during shipping. But they also removed the natural enzymes contained in all plant- and animal-derived foods. It's the enzymes that cause milk to sour and fruit to ripen. Knock out the enzymes, and everything lasts longer.

But at what price?

Howell went on to develop the *food enzyme concept*, which he originally published in a 1934 article entitled, "Are Food Enzymes Important in Digestion and Metabolism?"

Central to this new theory was the observation that foods in their raw, unprocessed and unpasteurized state are composed not only of protein, carbohydrates, fats, fibers, vitamins and minerals, but also enzymes, which assist in the digestion of these foods.

This early stage of digestion takes place in the food enzyme stomach, which exists as either a separate stomach or digestive compartment. In the cow, it's the first of four digestive compartments. In the bird, it's the crop—the pouch in the bird's gullet. In humans it's the upper "cardiac" portion of the stomach, where food is stored for 30 to 60 minutes, while hydrochloric acid is being created in the lower portion of the stomach as it expands to receive the meal.

Studies indicate that an average 60 percent of starches, 30 percent of proteins, and 10 percent of fats can be predigested by salivary enzymes and food enzymes before the stomach begins its own digestive processes—*if* the food enzymes haven't been destroyed prior to the foods being eaten.

Heat kills enzymes. In the case of pasteurization, Howell learned, heating milk to 190 degrees for 10 minutes, or to 160 degrees for 20 minutes, kills pretty much all of the "life element." In his own experiments, Dr. Howell found that immersion in water at 118 degrees Fahrenheit was capable of destroying enzymes within a half hour.

Slow or fast baking or broiling, stewing and frying all "destroy 100 percent of the enzymes in food," he wrote.

New technologies are now being used to breed enzymes and enzyme activity out of produce to further prolong shelf life.

Again, at what price?

The consequences for humans are an enzyme-deficient diet resulting in an overworked, enlarged pancreas—pound per pound of bodyweight the largest in the animal kingdom—incomplete digestion, and the recruitment of the immune system's enzyme-packing white blood cells to do digestive duties, resulting in intestinal autointoxication with even broader health implications.

In the introduction to Howell's book, *Enzyme Nutrition*, Stephan Blauer states Howell's conclusion that "many, if not all, degenerative diseases that humans suffer and die from are caused by the excessive use of enzyme-deficient cooked and processed foods."

This has been borne out in studies of Eskimo tribes subsisting on their traditional, enzyme raw diet. They remain free of cancer and heart disease compared to those who have adopted a cooked Western-style diet and have assimilated all the degenerative diseases associated with modern society—from cancer and heart disease to diabetes and arthritis.

Zoo studies cited by Howell reveal the same trend: Raw is good. Incorporating cooked and processed foods into wild animal diets, however, breeds the same array of diseases that plague humans.

Hence, we have Howell's strategy of incorporating food enzyme supplements as a means of bringing Nature's workers—the "life element"—back into the modern diet and achieving more healthful and complete digestion and delivery of nutrients to the body's cells.

This last point is key. It is generally assumed that the consumption of essential nutrients insures good health, which is not the case when the digestive system has been rendered incompetent by an enzyme-deficient diet.

In such a case, much of the nutritional content of the foods a person eats will not cross the intestinal barrier and reach the body's cells. In other words, a person can consume enough nutrients to run a power plant and still be energy deficient.

And that's what we're talking about. Energy.

It all comes down to more complete digestion.

How Digestion Works

Normal digestion begins in the mouth, with chewing, and with the release of enzymes by the salivary glands. Amylase from the parotid glands, protease from the submandibular glands, and lipase from the sublingual glands initiate starch, protein and fat digestion.

Food enzymes accomplish their predigestive work in the upper cardiac stomach, alongside the salivary enzymes, while the ingredients for hydrochloric acid (HCl) are coming together from the blood for the conversion of pepsinogen into protein-digesting pepsin.

Again, studies indicate that an average of 60 percent of starch, 30 percent of protein, and 10 percent of fat are predigested by salivary and food enzymes before the stomach begins its own digestive processes.

The next stage of digestion takes place in the small intestine, where the pancreas has prepared just the right proportion of protease, amylase and lipase enzymes to digest the meal entering from the stomach. This "recipe" is dictated by two hormones—secretin and cholecystokinin. Both hormones are activated by the partially digested food as it drops through the pyloric valve onto the wall of the upper portion of the small intestine, or the duodenum. These hormones are carried by the bloodstream to the pancreas, as well as to the biliary system of the liver.

Hence, whatever predigestion is accomplished prior to the food entering the small intestine is that much less effort for the overworked pancreas.

The final stage of carbohydrate digestion occurs in the middle portion of the small intestine, where microvilli—finger-like projections on the surface of epithelial cells—secrete lactase, maltase and sucrase. Insufficiency in any of these enzymes is capable of producing gas, bloating, and either painful diarrhea or constipation.

Nutrients (i.e., vitamins), and minerals (i.e., sodium, potassium), and water are absorbed in the small intestine. Residual minerals, water and undigested material are then passed on to the large intestine, which temporarily stores the undigested material, some of which is acted upon by resident bacteria.

It is estimated that between 70 percent and 90 percent of all cells in the human body are bacteria, living in the gastrointestinal tract. The maintenance of a normal bacterial flora is imperative for a healthy intestinal environment.

The colonic flora live in symbiosis with the human body, obtaining their nutrients from food particles that are not completely digested. These bacteria also play a very important role in preventing many pathogens from becoming established in the gut and causing disease.

When the body is unable to digest its food completely and eliminate the putrefying matter, the resident microorganisms can have both beneficial and detrimental effects. So-called "good bacteria" excrete acid waste, which improves bowel function; whereas, "bad bacteria" excrete alkaline waste, which results in constipation and an immune response to clean up the toxic mess.

So what are the consequences of incomplete digestion?

Food particles do not have to be digested down to their smallest size in order to be absorbed. So basically we're talking about two things:

1. Food particles not digested well enough to pass across the gut wall.

2. Food particles digested well enough to pass through the gut wall and into the blood, but not enough to be used by the body cells for energy production.

Food particles *not* digested well enough to be absorbed across the gut wall, mostly proteins and sugars, are acted upon by unfriendly bacteria in the last section of the small intestine (the ileum) and in the colon. The result is an overgrowth of unfriendly bacteria and the toxins they release, along with the accumulation of undigested food in the large intestine. The more putrefaction that is taking place, the more constipated a person becomes.

Toxic chemicals, including indican, are formed. These chemicals can irritate the mucosal barrier that protects the wall of the gastrointestinal tract. When the mucosal barrier is sufficiently compromised, the result is "leaky gut" syndrome. The integrity of the bowel itself becomes compromised in leaky gut syndrome, allowing partially digested food particles and bacterial endotoxins to leak through the gut into the lymphatics and the bloodstream.

These compounds can cause a number of inflammatory problems before they can be detoxified by the liver and eliminated. They can overwhelm weaker organs, producing pain and an inflammatory immune response.

This is why the body's ability to produce and maintain normal, healthy, well-nourished mucosal cells, to protect the walls of the gastrointestinal tract, is imperative.

When the mucosal barrier fails, the immune system is called into action. Certain white blood cells (T-cells) lining the mucosal barrier act to prevent toxic elements from crossing the barrier and entering the body. Other white blood cells hurry to clean up any area of inflammation caused by irritation.

When undigested food particles cross the intestinal wall, which has become inflamed and more permeable, antibodies created by leukocytes attach themselves to these particles to form what are called *circulating immune complexes*. Some of these complexes will be consumed by macrophages on the hunt, while others will continue to circulate until the blood or other extracellular fluids become overloaded and they begin settling on cell surfaces inside artery walls, in the joints, etc. Each cell, in turn, has its own little pocket of enzymes, called lysosomes, for dealing with material that falls out of circulation onto its surface. Unfortunately, inflammation and tissue destruction are an inevitable byproduct of this ongoing battle.

This immune response to digestive duties was first described by Rudolph Virchow, the father of cellular pathology, in 1897. Virchow considered digestive leukocytosis, or the sudden increase in the number of white blood cells following a meal, to be normal, because it occurred in all of his patients.

It was Dr. Paul Kouchakoff, in 1930, who demonstrated that there was nothing normal about digestive leukocytosis at all. His findings, drawn from thousands of blood tests, revealed that white blood cell counts go up after a person eats a meal consisting of enzyme-deficient cooked or processed foods—but not after a raw meal!

Kouchakoff was actually able to divide his findings into four distinct categories:

- Raw or frozen food produced no increase in the white blood cell count.
- Commonly cooked food caused mild leukocytosis.
- Pressure-cooked or canned food produced moderate white blood cell elevation.
- Human-made foods, which contain no food enzymes, caused severe leukocytosis. Carbonated beverages, alcohol, white sugar, flour and vinegar, were the biggest offenders.

Kouchakoff went so far as to prove that meat must be eaten raw to avoid leukocytosis, and that cured, salted, canned, and cooked meats brought on a violent reaction equivalent to the leukocytosis seen in poisoning.

The bottom line:
The human body needs food enzymes to predigest foods. When food enzymes are not present, the body must mobilize the immune system to complete the digestive process and clean up the resulting toxic mess.

With this in mind, it's no wonder that chronic degenerative diseases are not only increasing in the general population, but these diseases appear at earlier stages of life than ever before.

And so, as Doc Howell would say, we are not as healthy as we seem. We are a collection of diseases in progress, all stemming to a great extent from a digestive system rendered incompetent by an enzyme-deficient diet.

The other side of this coin is the impaired delivery of nutrients across an incompetent digestive system.

And so we come back to the energy needed by the 10 organ systems to maintain homeostasis and an overall healthy environment within the human body.

> **My plan was to devise a comprehensive diagnostic system for determining when to use which supplemental food enzyme, or enzyme combination, to relieve the symptoms being manifested by a body suffering from an apparent energy deficiency.**

I would use the methods taught to all health care providers, namely:

1. A careful case history, including past health problems, surgeries, and the use of over-the-counter and prescription medications.

2. Physical examination. It was here that I truly began to appreciate the key principles of my chiropractic education—its recognition that the body's structural and visceral components are inseparable parts of a whole and must be recognized and treated as such—with involuntary muscle contractions being the key. That's *if* I was to determine the source of a symptomatic complaint (SOS), and to plan a course of treatment for the patient.

3. Laboratory procedures. To establish a treatment plan and offer a prognosis to the patient, lab work was needed. Blood and urine testing, for example, were a means of ruling out pathology and irreparable damage, in which case the patient would be referred to the right health care provider for appropriate treatment. It's worth noting, however, that patients under medical care for a disease process, or recovering from a surgical procedure, need complete nutrition, including food enzymes, for restoration of normal body processes, as do "healthy individuals" who are only experiencing inconvenient symptoms.

And so my five years began, each case a lesson unto itself.

LESSON #1: Food Enzymes Can Move Essential Nutrients Past an Incompetent Digestive System.

The first such case was a woman in her late 50s who worked at the courthouse three doors down from my office in Forsyth. She had sought me out not as a chiropractor but specifically because she had heard that I was working with digestive enzymes. It was a small community and word was getting around.

She was a cancer survivor whose treatment had unfortunately involved the surgical removal of most of her stomach. Hence, there was no place to initiate digestion. She was receiving regular vitamin B12 injections and intravenous calcium drips, because her nutritional absorption was dramatically impaired, and she was slowly losing weight. She was down to 98 pounds when she came to see me, and she was desperate.

"If I lose two more pounds, I'm going to die!" she cried.

It probably wasn't true, but she was convinced she was going to die. I will never forget that.

It didn't matter what she ate, everything went right through her. Within minutes of eating she would have a bowel movement containing undigested food. She wanted to know if I could help her gain weight.

More and more, I would find myself the last refuge of desperate people who would come to me and say, 'I know you don't do this, but I have no place else to go. Would you at least try?'

What was I supposed to say to them? No?

I told her that I didn't know if I could help her because I had never worked with such a case. The only thing I knew for certain was that supplemental food enzymes worked in the stomach for an average of 45 minutes before her own digestive process would begin. Since most of her stomach had been removed, I just didn't know if the food enzymes would help.

And with no digestion taking place in the stomach, there were no hormonal signals going to the liver and pancreas telling them how to prepare for the meal coming down the digestive tract.

Forget the absence of food enzymes. Hers was as incompetent a digestive system as I was ever likely to encounter.

Nevertheless, she asked, and I agreed. She understood that we were taking at best "a shot in the dark."

I wound up cautiously giving her a mild predigestive formula consisting of protease, amylase, lipase and cellulase. Since I doubted the capsules would have enough time in her stomach to melt, I asked her to open them up and sprinkle the contents on her food. I figured that would at least give her a "puncher's chance," as they say in boxing lingo.

To make a long story short, it worked. With the food enzymes on board, her entire digestive process slowed down, and she began to gain weight. A few months later, her IV drips and vitamin B12 injections were discontinued.

The last time I saw her, 10 years later, she and her husband came to see me in Branson, where I was holding a seminar. She was still taking digestive enzyme supplements, and she was still healthy and enjoying life.

Never underestimate the power of enzymes.

LESSON #2: No Nutritional Supplement Can Replace Food Enzymes.

He was the kindest, gentlest man I ever met.

He was a cancer survivor in his early 70s. His treatment for lymphatic cancer had been successful, but all of the muscles on the right side of his neck had been surgically removed, leaving his head bent forward at the shoulders. He was unable to lay flat in bed.

He had not come to me for an adjustment, however. What brought him to me were the chronic abdominal pains and involuntary muscle contractions that occurred every time he ate, for many years.

He had been treated for chronic pancreatitis. The specialists at the University of Missouri had prescribed him pancreatic enzymes combined with a narcotic pain reliever. And yet, the abdominal pains continued to double him over, every time he ate.

He had come to me because he had heard I was working with enzymes.

I had instructed him to have something to eat before he came to the office, and the involuntary muscle contractions were palpable by the time I examined him. They were right in the upper part of the abdomen. I could feel it. I know where the pancreas is, where the liver and the spleen are. We're taught to palpate for signs of stress from these organs.

THE ENZYME ADVANTAGE

My examination and the urinalysis told me that I needed a formula more suited for protein and lipid digestion in his case, to take some of the workload off the pancreas and improve protein digestion and the flow of bile. He was all stopped up.

Two capsules with each meal did the trick. His pain stopped with the first meal. He called me on the phone from home.

It was all about predigestion.

This man's immediate relief from years of abdominal muscle contractions every time he ate proved to me beyond a doubt the ability of food enzymes to predigest foods. Predigesting the foods he was eating relieved the burden on his overworked pancreas.

That had been my strategy from the beginning, and it worked.

LESSON #3: Are You Eating to Your Genetic Strength or Your Genetic Weakness?

The sickest patients often have the best diet. This is true because the advice they receive is based on the nutrient content of various foods, not on their ability to digest these foods adequately.

Raw fruits and vegetables and whole grains are touted by most nutrition books as being healthy for you, but this is true only if you can digest them adequately. If you are already having unresolved health problems, consuming foods you are not able to digest adequately will only compound these problems by draining more of your body's much-needed energy.

Indeed, the sickest people I have seen are those who are eating whole grains and vegetables and are unable to digest them.

What makes whole grains and vegetables difficult to digest?

In the case of fiber-rich vegetables and fruits, it's all about cellulose. All fibrous foods are covered with cellulose. The human body does not make cellulase, the enzyme needed to digest cellulose. The only source of cellulase for human digestion is in the vegetable itself—the food enzyme—which is not enough to do the entire digestive job. And now, with food enzymes being genetically manipulated from produce to prolong shelf life, there are even less enzymes available. Cellulase in these fiber-rich vegetables must be either cooked or chewed off. This is why people who do not chew their foods adequately wind up with gas and bloating when they eat raw, high-fiber produce.

Whole grains, such as wheat, oats, barley, maize, and quinoa, are another story. Grains like wheat and oats are not eaten raw. They are cooked. Amylase in the small intestine digests the starches, which produces the sugar, maltose, which is then converted by maltase into glucose, the body's primary source of energy.

If you can't convert maltose into glucose, you've got problems. This is often referred to as gluten intolerance.

People who are sucrose intolerant cannot breakdown cane or beet sugar into glucose and fructose.

People who are lactose intolerant don't have enough lactase to convert lactose from milk into its active energy products—glucose and galactose, which are bound together.

Depending on the sugar involved, these cases result in gas and bloating and diarrhea, or constipation.

The bottom line: Gas, bloating, constipation and diarrhea are signs that the body is struggling to digest the food it cannot digest.

It's important to note that no one is completely lactose intolerant and no one can drink all the milk or eat all the ice cream they want, just like no one is totally gluten intolerant or can eat all the wheat they want. We're all somewhere in between on a scale of zero to 100. In any situation, it's all about how much you consume compared to the amount of necessary enzyme your body can produce.

Gas and bloating result anytime you have a digestive problem of any type. This is why doctors have such difficulty sorting out exactly what a patient's problem is—whether their symptoms are coming from the gallbladder, the stomach, the pancreas or the jejunum.

It certainly made for a difficult five years for me; I had nowhere to go to get this information. It was a learning curve, but a lot of what I had been taught from books was not totally correct—because of the absence of the enzyme factor.

That was the missing link—enzymes.

The worst case of food intolerance that ever came through my door was a lady who had driven to see me from Maine. She'd come down with her daughter, who was a nurse. At the time of her visit, she was down to eating just two foods—baked potatoes and cooked beets. That was all she could eat.

She wanted desperately to eat the perfect diet—whole grains and high-fiber fruits and vegetables. But she couldn't digest them. They gave her terrible gas, bloating and diarrhea. The same happened when she tried to eat dairy products.

Basically, she couldn't digest sugars, which was a major-league problem. She had an advanced digestive enzyme deficiency, most of it in the jejunum, because that's where sugars are digested.

She just didn't have the enzymes.

Chapter 3—Action

My first task in helping her was to figure out what was in beets and baked potatoes that digested easily. There were no enzymes; they had been cooked out.

Beets contain protein, betaine and sulfur. So she could handle things like that. And they don't contain fiber. All the nutrition books say cooking is a digestive aid because it breaks down fiber, which is true.

So the only thing she seemed to be able to digest was protein.

However, a careful case history—physical examination, urinalysis and blood work—told me that this lady was actually protein deficient.

I needed to turn her mind around and get her eating towards her genetic strength. The first thing I did was tell her what I had learned and suggest that she stay away from high-fiber fruits and vegetables for a while (which she was already doing out of necessity), and eat more protein. To prove my point, I sent her to a local restaurant and asked her to order a hamburger without the bun.

"Just eat the hamburger," I told her.

Her daughter, the nurse, had a fit. "You can't do that to her!" she said.

"According to my findings," I replied, "that's what she can digest."

So they went out to lunch, with an enzyme supplement to help out, and when she came back she was literally beaming.

"I never thought I could eat a meal like that!" she said. "I feel wonderful!"

Basically, she found out she could digest protein. It was the sugars and fiber that were affecting her.

With time, we were able to modify her diet. I got her to eat more protein. It was okay for to have eggs and meat. But she needed to stay away from high-fiber foods. There are lots of fruits and vegetables that are not high in fiber. And I gave her an enzyme supplement containing cellulase to digest any fiber that she might take in.

"And obviously we want you to stay away from whole grains and milk and dairy products," I told her.

The good news is, we expanded her diet to more than cooked beets and baked potatoes.

In time, she was able to broaden her diet somewhat, with the help of supplemental enzymes for predigestion, but she continued eating towards her genetic strength—protein—to supply her body with the energy it needed.

LESSON #4: Concentrated Vitamins and Minerals Are Not Food!

Another important patient during my five-year learning curve was a woman who had undergone bladder repair surgery. She had bleeding problems early in her surgery, and because of her religious beliefs, the doctors had to halt the procedure and close her up after they stopped the bleeding. They knew a blood transfusion would not be an option if the bleeding had continued or gotten worse.

The next day, the doctors ran blood tests and found her to be incredibly anemic. So they placed her on a ferris sulfate, a pharmaceutical iron supplement. The problem is, pharmaceutical supplements, including concentrated vitamins and minerals, are not food. They're chemicals. And if the body cannot absorb and use them, a patient has a problem. No matter how much goes in, the body simply can't use it. This is what happened in this woman's case.

For six weeks, the doctors were unable to raise her blood iron count.

The secret here is that iron, as a mineral, is totally dependent on protein for its digestion, absorption, transportation and use. If you're protein deficient, you don't have anything that will carry that iron and use it, even if you dump a load of it into the digestive tract. The body simply can't use it. Iron has to be absorbed on protein. It has to be carried through the blood on protein. It has to be used by the red blood cells. Hemoglobin is an iron-containing protein molecule used in the transport of oxygen to the body cells.

It made sense that this lady was protein deficient. And that's what my physical examination told me. She had involuntary muscle contractions around her spleen, in the left flank area. That told me her spleen was the organ that was struggling.

There are three things that the spleen does. Essentially, it tells the bone marrow when to send it more red blood cells, or white blood cells, or more platelets.

Well, she wasn't running a fever, she wasn't short on white blood cells; she wasn't bruising, so she wasn't deficient in platelets. She was deficient in iron, so she was deficient in red blood cells, and that spells protein deficiency. Because that's what red blood cells do—they carry hemoglobin, which is a protein molecule, which is bound to iron.

She was protein deficient. Her blood tests confirmed that. So the first step was to fix her protein deficiency, which should result in more iron being absorbed.

As it happened, I had just read a study that had come out of Penn State University that said that the body was more capable of using iron out of foods, like spinach and liver, than it was using iron out of iron supplements.

And so we put her on an herbal formula high in natural iron containing Pau D'Arco, Yellow Dock, Echinacea and Astragalus. This formula was blended and encapsulated with a broad food enzyme mixture that emphasized protease, to predigest the protein that would transport the iron past her incompetent digestive system and for absorption into her body and her cells.

Two weeks later, her blood iron count was up to normal.

LESSON #5: The Power of Nutrition—With Enzymes

Once again, the person in my office had not come to me for chiropractic care.

This was an elderly woman who had been living alone since her husband had died. She was a sweet lady, a rural farm girl with a full head of white hair. She had come to me because she had been experiencing unrelenting trembling for some time, to the point where she was unable to hold her hand still enough to eat soup. She had already been through a thorough medical examination that had ruled out Parkinson's disease or any other disease pathology, and they assigned her problem simply to old age.

Her neighbors had convinced her to see me, because they heard mine was not a typical chiropractic office—that I was working with enzymes. She nevertheless doubted I would be able to help her. She had reached a point of despair.

I examined her, looking for pinched nerves or anything that might account for her trembling. I found nothing. But in the course of my examination, and in the blood testing and urinalysis, it became obvious that she might be very fat or lipid deficient.

The involuntary muscle contractions were in her lower abdomen, suggesting to me that she had a possible problem in female hormone production, as well as difficulty digesting lipids, leading to a lipid deficiency.

Hormones, particularly reproductive hormones, require lipids. As noted earlier, when the body is under stress, the brain instructs all body cells to switch from glucose to lipids for energy. As a result, the body lacks adequate lipids to make hormones.

Chapter 3—Action

Even though you're an 80-year-old woman, you still need hormones to some extent. The balance between estrogen and progesterone still needs to be maintained. Things change during menopause, but hormone production is not turned off.

Lipids are also needed to maintain the protective myelin sheath that covers the axons that connect the body's nerve cells, enabling communications between nerve cells throughout the body and the central nervous system.

It also followed that she would be deficient in fat soluble vitamins.

With all this in mind, I gave her herbal formulas high in lipids—wheat germ, which contains fat soluble vitamins, lipids and phospholipids, and I gave her artichoke extract and lecithin, a phospholipid. I did not give her oil, because if a person can't digest fat, there's no point in pouring oil into them.

I basically gave her herbal formulas high in lipids and the enzymes to digest those herbs—mostly lipase, along with protease, amylase and cellulase.

Because she'd had this problem for quite a while, I told her I was going to give her a higher dose than I normally would, to get her started.

And because she lived out in the country, transportation was a problem. She thought she would be able to make it back in a month. So I gave her explicit instructions about tapering off as needed.

I told her to start by taking four capsules with each meal. It wouldn't be too long before this dose would be too high for her. She would know this when she began feeling full after taking the capsules. When this happened, I told her to reduce her dose from four capsules to three, and finally to two capsules.

"I'm going to trust you to cut down your own dosage," I told her, "so you don't have to keep coming to town."

> **Food *for* Thought**
>
> **The ancients had it right.
> Maintaining balance—homeostasis—was the key.**

Give the body what it needs at the first sign of symptoms and it will heal itself, before full-blown disease develops.

It's all about prevention.

She didn't change her diet.

A month later she was back in my office. I was making rounds, from one treatment room to the next. When I opened the door to her room, she was sitting on the table. She held her arms out in front of her. There was no shaking.

"I'm so proud of you," she said.

I still tear up at the thought of it.

* * *

And enzymes were the means of delivering that nutrition

Those five years were an affirmation of what my healing art had taught me—that the structural and visceral aspects of the human body cannot be separated. Homeostasis is a two-sided phenomenon. The visceral side involves the maintenance of constant conditions within the extracellular fluids, while the structural side is the body's need to maintain itself against the constant pull of gravity.

Consider scoliosis, whereby the curvature of the spine impinges on the lung's ability to expand, and patients become acidic because they hold carbon dioxide.

It doesn't matter what position the body is in—a person can be standing upright or lying down, on the back or on the side. These two factors—the visceral and the structural—are constantly at play.

Chapter 3—Action

Maintaining homeostasis in the extracellular fluid and opposing the pull of gravity on the human body is a 24/7 effort. And it takes energy to do this—a continual source of energy.

When the person with orthostatic hypotension stands up, they experience light-headedness, dizziness, perhaps even confusion. Why? A change in position is supposed to stimulate the flow of a hormone from the adrenal glands to elevate blood pressure. If this does not occur, the blood does not get into the brain and the person becomes dizzy. It's the body trying to catch up with the change that's been made against gravity.

Treating the symptom without addressing the underlying cause is an ongoing exercise in futility.

> **Energy is key.**
> **If a person is not able to create an adequate supply of glucose from carbohydrate, the body must get its energy from someplace else. Such patients begin to become protein deficient. This is why patients under chronic stress—be it structural, visceral or emotional—are all protein deficient.**

The last resort is to turn stored fat into energy.

So the question becomes: Are a patient's symptoms coming from a carbohydrate, protein or lipid deficiency?

And are the symptoms structural or visceral in origin?

Regardless, there will be tell-tale muscle contractions. And so my chiropractic education pointed me toward diagnosis, not just therapy. Because the brain does not separate structure from visceral. Everything is connected by nervous system function.

I became a doctor looking for causes, not simply treating symptoms. So get out your mirrors.

Food *for* Thought

In the next three chapters, we'll be making rounds, taking a close look at the three energy deficiencies that plague all of us—carbohydrate, protein and fat deficiencies.

Part Two—What Is Your Deficiency?

"It really isn't rocket science. What do you crave? But besides increasing ingestion of what you crave, improve its digestion as well."

—Howard F. Loomis, Jr., D.C., F.I.A.C.A.

"I was a vegetarian for 10 years and a pescetarian for eight. Then I woke up one day when I was 29 and craved red meat. I'm a big believer in listening to my body's cravings."

—Chelsea Clinton

Chapter 4

Carbohydrate: The Perfect Fuel

So it's all about energy and the maintenance of normal function.

It's about maintaining homeostasis in the midst of ongoing challenges, whether the challenge is biochemical in nature, or the constant force of gravity acting on the body as it makes its way through the physical universe, or the emotional challenge that occurs when the IRS comes knocking.

It doesn't matter whether the challenge/stress is structural or visceral, mechanical or emotional, acute or chronic. The body is going to need energy to deal with it.

It's that simple.

And that energy is delivered to body cells in the form of nutrition.

Not all organs require the same nutrients.

The heart, for example, in addition to fatty acids, needs alkaline minerals, like potassium, to maintain its rhythm. And because the heart is a muscle, it needs B vitamins to remain healthy and perform its work.

The stomach, the lung and the urinary bladder have protective mucosal linings. They need to be able to create mucus. Useful in this regard, besides a generous helping of escargot with buttery garlic sauce, would be herbs the body can digest to feed the cells that produce mucus—e.g., slippery elm, marshmallow root and okra.

When it comes to meeting the body's energy needs, however, vitamins and minerals, while essential, cannot be converted directly into energy. They are building blocks, pure and simple.

The human body has three sources of energy: carbohydrates, protein and fat, and the body uses them in that order.

The body prefers carbohydrates as its primary source of glucose to supply energy. When the body runs out of carbohydrates, it turns to protein as its second source of glucose, and finally to stored fat.

Why the preference for carbohydrate? Because it's a high-energy food that is easily converted into energy by the cells. However, carbohydrates are not stored widely in the body—only in the liver and the muscles, as an emergency source of energy. While muscles store glucose, in the form of glycogen, this can only be used by the muscles in the event of a "fight or flight" situation, where there is an acute demand for energy to meet an emergency.

When the body does not have enough carbohydrates, it turns to protein. Each cell hoards protein in the form of amino acids, which they can use to repair themselves, or to reproduce. When the

Chapter 4—Carbohydrate: The Perfect Fuel

carbohydrate supply is exhausted and an alternate source of energy is needed, the brain instructs cells to send their amino acids to the liver to be converted to glucose. This means that anybody who is under stress for any length of time—be it biochemical, structural or emotional—is going to become protein deficient.

Only when the body is protein deficient will it turn to lipids, or fats.

While every cell in the body is capable of using fat for energy, if the need arises, the brain is not able to convert fat to glucose fast enough to keep working. It needs high octane fuel. This is why the brain gets first dibs on all available glucose.

Again, it's all about energy, which brings us back to enzymes.

* * *

I began to realize early on that a great many of my patients were suffering from chronic energy deficiencies.

What I found in patient after patient, in addition to their primary reason for seeking treatment, were universal complaints of fatigue, or simply being tired.

This, in fact, is the most common symptom expressed by patients to health care providers.

In addition, as a chiropractor, I also found in patients complaining of fatigue involuntary muscle contractions across the top of the shoulders and commonly—but not always—up the neck to the head, and extending down the spine between the shoulder blades.

From the time I entered practice, and for the 12 years before I began using enzymes, I had treated many patients suffering from "muscle tension headaches" by adjusting those areas. I always managed to get excellent short-term results. But in those patients with chronic muscle tension headaches, the problem invariably returned.

Because the problem was not structural but visceral.

And, I would soon realize, it had to do with energy, or a lack of it, often as a result of inadequate dietary intake and/or inadequate digestion.

I knew that the digestive organs received their neurological innervations from the middle thoracic spine, between the shoulder blades. Hence the involuntary muscle contractions and chronic headaches.

As mentioned in Chapter 2, I had no success using over-the-counter vitamin and mineral preparations by themselves. But when I had food enzymes to assist with predigestion, my entire practice changed. I could now not only treat the chronic headache complaints stemming from digestive stress, but I could also determine which part of the patient's diet they had difficulties digesting. With this information, I was able to change the patient's diet and use food enzyme supplementation to provide the specific nutrition needed to energize the struggling organ or organs.

And I had found an answer to chronic shoulder problems where there was no traumatic injury or tissue damage. Many of those shoulder and arm problems emanate from the bowel, due to involuntary muscle contractions in the lower abdomen. These muscle contractions can cause compensatory postural changes as the body attempts to remain aligned against gravity.

> **Looking back, I had been given an incredible gift from Dr. Howell and his dedicated efforts to prove that food enzymes are essential nutrients despite their systematic removal from our diets through cooking, in order to extend shelf life to provide for an increasingly industrialized world.**

Chapter 4—Carbohydrate: The Perfect Fuel

I could have simply stopped with this knowledge and maintained a very busy practice until I retired. However, I soon came to realize that there was much more to be learned as the energy-depleting effects of an enzyme-deficient diet became more and more apparent.

It starts with the brain.

When it comes to maintaining homeostasis, the hypothalamus rules. The gland responds to signals from various tissues and organs via the autonomic nervous system, which has both sympathetic and parasympathetic controls. While the sympathetic nervous system is responsible for mobilizing the body for fight-or-flight response, both systems are constantly involved in maintaining homeostasis.

The autonomic nervous system is used to maintain balance. If the hypothalamus wants the heart to run faster, it may send the signal through the sympathetic system; if it wants the heart to run slower, it may send the signal through the parasympathetic system.

When the body is in a fight-or-flight situation, the sympathetic system kicks in, increasing blood flow to the muscles, while reducing blood flow to organs not needed to meet the challenge—in particular the digestive organs.

Both of these systems are intimately related to nutrition. It's a balance between calcium and potassium. For example, if you are deficient in potassium, you'll have symptoms of autonomic imbalance because the parasympathetic system can't do its job. If you are deficient in protein and calcium, you will have symptoms of autonomic imbalance because the sympathetic system can't do its job.

Now the critical point. When asked what the first response is when the door opens and a bear enters, most health care practitioners will say it's a fight-or-flight response on the part of the sympathetic nervous system. In fact, that is the second response. The first response is the hypothalamus deciding if it has enough glucose to produce the energy to meet the challenge, whether that be to run or fight or whatever.

Does the body have the energy to meet the challenge?

That's the bottom line. It's one thing for the brain to send a signal to an organ, and it's quite another thing for that organ to respond. Because that response requires energy.

It's at this point that a person begins to experience symptoms, when there's a lack of energy.

The symptom is actually a distress signal—an SOS—sent by an organ unable to respond to the brain's instructions due to an energy shortage. The good news is, if you can find the Source of Stress, the SOS, and give that organ what it needs, you've got it made.

The general symptoms of an ongoing energy deficiency include: headache; heartburn; indigestion; gas and bloating; infrequent bowel movements (constipation); frequent, soft bowel movements; anxiety; irritability; difficulty falling asleep; and waking after a few hours, unable to return to sleep.

We're not talking about fight-or-flight challenges—i.e., that bear entering the room, or other such emergent situation. This is about the insidious long-term effects associated with chronic energy deficiency, resulting from chronic stress, which sets off a step-by-step cascade of physiological events that is as common as life itself.

* * *

Recalling Hans Selye's research, which received multiple Nobel Prize nominations, stress is not a vague undefinable term having only to do with our being unloved, underworked and underpaid. Rather, the human body responds to any kind of stress—be it mechanical, chemical or emotional—in a very specific, predictable way.

Selye called this response the "general adaptation syndrome."

It's all about stimulus and alarm, resistance and compensation by the body that we don't even notice until exhaustion sets in and symptoms appear that can lead to disease and degeneration.

It begins when the body realizes that it does not have adequate glucose to meet the energy demands of the stress. This sets off a chain of very specific physiological events, driven by the sympathetic nervous system.

It doesn't matter if it's acute stress arising from a fight-or-flight situation, stress resulting from a structural or biochemical issue, emotional stress, the unrelenting stress one experiences as a caregiver for an elderly parent, or a parent with a difficult child, or an executive running a company.

Stress is stress. The sympathetic response is always the same. It's just a matter of degree.

Here's how it plays out:

- **Increased Arterial Pressure.**

  The first stage of any emergent fight-or-flight response involves increasing the heart rate and a constriction of the blood vessels, resulting in an increase in blood pressure, resulting in more blood to the extremities as opposed to the core of the body.

The same is true with chronic stress. Health care providers: How many of your patients have high blood pressure?

- **Increased Blood Flow to Active Muscles Combined with Decreased Blood Flow to Organs Not Needed for Rapid Activity.**
  This means decreased blood flow to the digestive system, digestive symptoms, and involuntary muscle contractions, as the digestive organs struggle to do their jobs.

- **Increased Rates of Cellular Metabolism Throughout the Body.**
  This means that the cells are consuming more nutrition and putting out more waste, which places a greater challenge on organ systems responsible for maintaining homeostasis.

As the taxes go up with the increasing effort to maintain homeostasis, and nutritional fuel becomes less available, symptoms appear: joint pain, increased heat, swelling, redness, pain and involuntary muscle contraction.

Those organs responsible for waste removal are heavily taxed. How many people today suffer from unexplained kidney, lung and skin problems?

Increased cellular activity is driven by the thyroid's production of thyroxine. This hormone does not grow on trees. Its manufacture involves attaching four iodine molecules to a large protein molecule, which must then incubate for seven to eight days. Under constant demand, supplies of protein, calcium and magnesium needed to produce thyroxine can run out.

It's at this point that the overstressed caregiver's metabolic rate slows down and they feel like they have no energy. The synthetic hormone Synthroid may be prescribed.

If one could just relieve the stress and nourish the thyroid, there would be less need for this medication.

- **Increased Glycolysis in Muscle.**

    Muscles convert their stored glycogen to glucose to meet their own increased energy needs, which means it won't be available for the rest of the body. Glycogen stored in the liver can be released into the blood in times of stress, and that is made available to the brain, reproductive system, and the eyes, none of which can convert fat to glucose fast enough to maintain normal function. As the body's organs struggle to perform their jobs in the midst of the energy shortage, involuntary muscle contractions result, causing structural misalignments.

    This is where the chiropractor comes in, diagnosing and treating structural symptoms of visceral origin.

- **Increased Blood Clotting Ability.**

    This is why people are advised to take low-dose aspirin daily. Indeed, how many people are taking so-called "blood thinners" to reduce their risk of heart attacks and strokes?

    Actually, the concept of blood thinning is erroneous. One cannot thin the blood without losing homeostasis. The purpose of daily aspirin is to break up these blood clots as they form.

    Another byproduct of chronic stress is the backing up of excessive cholesterol into the blood. In an unstressed body, cholesterol is destined for the bile.

    How many millions are on statins today?

- **Increased Conversion of Glycogen to Glucose by the Liver.**

    When glucose levels fall, the liver converts glycogen to glucose and releases it into the blood for transport to the brain and the reproductive system. When the body is under chronic stress, a person's energy bank account can become overdrawn and they can begin having difficulty making it through the day, both physically and mentally.

One can literally lose their ability to think clearly. In fact, the stress of continual mental activity itself is enough to bring about a body-wide energy crisis. Physiological studies conducted on Grand Master Chess players have shown that they use as much energy as a boxer fighting 10 rounds!

- **Increased Conversion of Cellular Amino Acids to Glucose by the Liver.**
  When the body runs out of glucose, it turns to protein contained in body cells in the form of amino acids. In the next chapter, we'll be talking about the symptoms of protein deficiency and its effect on the body's ability to repair damaged tissues.

- **Increased Mental Activity.**
  People doing mental work will run out of glucose more quickly under stress. Stress is hardest on heavy thinkers, particularly as it affects the reproductive system.

Compare this to the physical laborer whose muscles are breaking down glycogen and using it for the work. In this case, the brain is not as heavily taxed.

So the mental laborer is using up glucose faster than the physical laborer.

Chapter 4—Carbohydrate: The Perfect Fuel

The list goes on. ...

When tissues don't have adequate energy to respond, the pituitary is stimulated to release ACTH, which causes the adrenal cortex to release cortisol. It is released in response to stress and a low level of blood glucose. Cortisol's functions generally are to increase blood sugar through the conversion of protein in the liver (gluconeogenesis) to glycogen and then glucose, and to aid the metabolism of fat, protein and carbohydrate.

Before this occurs, the body suffers from symptoms of inflammation—heat, redness, swelling, pain. As the sediment increases, the patient may be diagnosed with rheumatoid arthritis, gout, or even asthma, all of which are treated medically with cortisone-related drugs as cortisol replacements.

How many of these cases can be prevented from reaching the state of chronic degeneration by identifying the specific stress that is leading to the decline and taking the right steps?

Selye had it right. It all comes down to energy, and nutrition is the key. A stress situation, he observed, will continue without issue as long as the flow of nutrition is maintained and the waste products produced by the affected organs/tissues are transported away and not allowed to accumulate.

It comes down to each organ having the energy to do its job.

And so we turn to the body's preferred source of energy: carbohydrates.

Nutrition books agree that a healthy diet consists of liberal helpings of fresh fruits and vegetables. They are the highest of any foods in carbohydrates. They also supply essential vitamins, especially vitamins B and C, and alkaline minerals—sodium, potassium and magnesium. These minerals, along with vitamins B and C, are all needed for the conversion of carbohydrates to energy.

An absence of fresh fruits and vegetables in one's diet is not a healthy thing. The same is true when these foods are consumed but not adequately digested for use by the body's cells, due to a shortage of digestive enzymes.

It's also true that consuming simple carbohydrates, like white flour or simple sugars, can actually lead to a depletion of these essential vitamins and minerals, as we will see.

So it doesn't matter whether you're not eating fresh fruits and vegetables, or not digesting them, or you're consuming copious amounts of simple sugars.

It all leads to the same set of problems.

So let's talk about how we digest carbohydrates and what a carbohydrate deficiency looks like.

Time to get out your mirrors.

So what is a carbohydrate, besides being the best source of energy a body can hope for?

Carbohydrate is composed of fiber, starch and simple sugars.

There are two types of dietary fiber—insoluble and soluble.

Insoluble fiber does not dissolve in water and cannot be digested. It is metabolically inert and provides bulking for bowel movements by absorbing water as they move through the digestive system. That's all insoluble fiber is good for—pulling water out and creating bulk in the stool.

Sources of insoluble fiber include: whole wheat, whole grains, wheat bran, corn bran, seeds, nuts, barley, brown rice, bulgur,

Chapter 4—Carbohydrate: The Perfect Fuel

zucchini, celery, broccoli, cabbage, onions, tomatoes, carrots, cucumbers, green beans, dark leafy vegetables, raisins, grapes, and fruit and root vegetable skins. It has often been reported that all fiber is indigestible. (This is not entirely the case with soluble fiber, which dissolves in water and is readily acted upon by the microorganisms residing in the colon.) This action tends to slow the movement of waste material through the colon. It also results in the production of gases and other byproducts, many of which must be absorbed by the body, transported to the liver to be detoxified, and then excreted through the kidneys.

This often results in symptoms of so-called "leaky gut."

Sources of soluble fiber include: oatmeal, oat cereal, oat bran, apples, peanuts, lentils, oranges, pears, strawberries, nuts, flaxseeds, beans, dried peas, blueberries, cucumbers, celery and carrots.

While the body does not make an enzyme to digest fiber, cellulase is present in any fresh fruit or vegetable with fiber content. This food enzyme is critically important because fibrous fruits and vegetables are covered with a layer of cellulose that must be either chewed or cooked off, or one will develop gas when eating raw food.

Cellulase does digest soluble fiber, which is a good source of glucose and short chain fatty acids, which are an important source of energy for colonic cells, and thus contribute to overall colon health. Short chain fatty acids have also been shown to have anti-carcinogenic and anti-inflammatory properties, as well as being essential in the production of hormones, maintaining healthy skin and keeping cell membranes permeable.

Let's turn to starch.

Starch is a form of carbohydrate that consists of a large number of glucose molecules—an excellent source of energy. These molecules are referred to as polysaccharides and are the most common carbohydrate found in fruits and vegetables.

The human body can store starch in the form of glycogen, in the liver, and easily convert it to glucose when needed to maintain homeostasis.

Glycogen stored in muscles is only used for physical activity.

Studies indicate that 40 percent to 80 percent of starches can be digested within 15 minutes of ingestion. This occurs before the stomach acid begins its own digestive process. Interestingly, people who consistently eat a diet of fresh fruits and vegetables produce more salivary amylase than those who do not.

The combined digestive efforts of salivary and pancreatic amylase result in the production of simple sugars. There still remains, however, one more vital digestive step in the release of glucose from our foods that can be used to produce energy, and this is where the rubber hits the road, so to speak.

Pancreatic amylase cannot complete carbohydrate digestion. It only breaks down the large carbohydrate (polysaccharide) molecules to two smaller disaccharide sugar molecules, and this is where a lot of digestive problems occur. These are molecules bonded together as follows: lactose (from dairy products), maltose (from grains), and sucrose (from white sugar or flour). These sugars must be digested further in order to be available to the body as nutrients.

This final digestive step is performed by the small fibers in the wall of the second portion of the small intestine, or the jejunum. It is here that Nature's workers—the enzymes that break sugars down (lactase, maltase and sucrase)—are secreted and finish the digestion of carbohydrate to glucose, fructose and galactose. If adequate amounts of these disaccharides cannot be made, or if excessive amounts of these sugars are consumed, then problems result in bowel movements.

Chapter 4—Carbohydrate: The Perfect Fuel

Further, lactose from dairy and maltose from grains, in the undigested state, create painful gas and bloating, as well as frequent soft bowel movements and diarrhea.

Likewise, undigested sucrose cannot be turned into glucose and will also cause painful gas and bloating, as well as infrequent bowel movements and often constipation.

And so, a person can eat the healthiest diet, with a full complement of fresh fruits and vegetables, and still be carbohydrate deficient. Because what isn't adequately digested will not make it to the body cells where it is needed to create energy, and it can raise havoc in the digestive system.

Then there's the impact of simple sugars—i.e., white flour and sucrose. Their manufacture involves the removal not only of the enzymes that would aid in their digestion but also the essential vitamins (B and C) and minerals (sodium, potassium) needed to convert sugar into energy.

Hence, a diet high in refined sugar at the expense of fresh fruits and vegetables will produce deficiencies in these vital nutrients as the body scavenges for them to turn sugars into energy.

Refined carbs also make for a less than desirable fuel because they burn too fast and leave the brain crying for more an hour later.

Today it is estimated that the average person consumes 100 pounds of sugar per year. In 1984, 45 percent of the calories in the diet came from carbohydrate. In 1900, that percentage was 56 percent. However, in the same time period, the amount of sugar intake increased by more than 50 percent, while complex carbohydrates decreased by the same amount.

So what does a carbohydrate deficiency look like?

One has only to look at the early days of the low-carb diet, which was intended to induce a carbohydrate deficiency by avoiding starches, and white flour and sugar, so the body would burn stored fat for energy. This worked quite well, but it produced ketones, a waste product that accumulates to greatly acidify the body. It also resulted in fatigue, dehydration and loss of energy. And it wasn't as effective as originally hoped, because the body is going to store more fat anyway. That's its reserve energy account, its port of last resort.

I saw a lot of people on the low-carb diet in my practice. They gradually became dehydrated and tended towards constipation and became calcium deficient with long-term use.

A total lack of carbohydrate in the diet can cause symptoms similar to those seen in starvation. And you don't have good waste removal. You just gradually begin to waste away, as if you were in a concentration camp.

While we know that carbohydrate is a dietary essential, we do not know how much is needed. But diets with as little as 60 grams of carbohydrate will prevent the symptoms of starvation. Most authorities feel it is prudent not to go below 100 grams per day.

And yet, carbohydrate deficiency is quite common. One can view its symptoms from a diet or digestive perspective.

From the dietary perspective:

This includes people who are not consuming enough carbohydrate to supply the body with energy, people who are not adequately digesting what they take in, and people who are consuming too much in the way of simple sugars, causing the body to use up its store of essential vitamins and alkaline minerals, reducing its ability to convert glucose into energy.

Chapter 4—Carbohydrate: The Perfect Fuel

The dietary symptoms of a carbohydrate deficiency include:

- **Dry Mouth, Nose or Eyes.** When you are carbohydrate deficient, your body loses water. It's that simple.

- **Muscle Weakness.** A reduced ability to exercise because the muscles lack stored glycogen.

- **One is Easily Startled.** This has to do with the alkaline mineral deficiency—potassium in particular—that occurs when too little carbohydrate is consumed, or too much simple sugar. Recent studies have shown that the potassium channels have a calming influence on the nerves, and they work "like shock absorbers, holding back sodium channel activity for a period after each nerve impulse."

- **Inability to Concentrate.** Not enough glucose for the brain. Pure and simple.

- **Difficulty Swallowing and Voice Affected by Stress.** This is often a sign of the salivary glands struggling to produce enough enzymes. And it brings up a fascinating story which goes back to when I first began formulating enzyme products for health care practitioners.

I was interested in understanding the use of amylase for digesting starch, or polysaccharides. I was aware that amylase was secreted by the parotid gland in the mouth. I also knew that vegetarians secreted more amylase than non-vegetarians. And I knew that involuntary muscle contractions will occur under the jaw when a patient had a sore throat or swollen tonsils.

However, when I began noticing such involuntary muscle contractions in the absence of a sore throat or swollen tonsils, I suspected that it might be a visceral issue, related to a struggling salivary gland. So I conducted a clinical trial involving a dozen such patients, giving them amylase supplements to take some of the workload off what I suspected was a stressed parotid gland.

And it worked. It relieved the muscle contractions in all of the patients, with a surprise added benefit in one.

This was a lady in her mid-40s. She was a very pleasant, laid back woman who spoke slowly and deliberately. She lived with her family in the Forsyth area and had come to me for a lower back problem which I corrected with adjustment.

However, as I was palpating various areas of her body for involuntary muscle contractions, I came across several hard nodules under her jaw. She told me she didn't have any problems there—no swollen tonsils, no sore throat, etc.

"But now that you're poking on it, it is a little sore," she said.

Usually, it's assumed that such bumps in that area are swollen lymph nodes.

I told her that I was developing this amylase formula and asked her if she would care to take part in a clinical trial.

She said she'd be happy to, and she took a bottle home with her.

I didn't hear from her for two or three months, when she came back for another adjustment for her back. I had forgotten about her nodules and was about to leave the treatment room when she said, "Oh, by the way, doctor, do you remember those capsules you gave me?" I said yes, and she said, "Well, I didn't call you back because I wasn't sure they were working until my friends and family started noticing the difference in my speech."

That's when I noticed she was talking less slowly.

It turned out she had had a speech impediment going back as far as she could remember.

Chapter 4—Carbohydrate: The Perfect Fuel

"I thought it was because I'm Polish and from Chicago," she said.

Well, the nodules were gone, and so was this lady's speech impediment, which I surmised was the result of the muscle contractions restricting her tongue's range of motion.

I'm not suggesting that amylase supplements are an effective remedy for speech impediments. However, they can be an effective means of relaxing involuntary muscle contractions related to salivary organs struggling to secrete amylase for carbohydrate digestion.

Any further benefit, as they say, is just icing on the cake.

Now for the digestive perspective.

There's nothing so subtle about symptoms of carbohydrate deficiencies relating to actual digestive issues.

These include:

- **History of Reactive Hypoglycemia**—a drop in blood sugar in the hours following a meal. This is an almost allergic reaction to carbohydrates, in particular whole grains and dairy products, suffered by the gluten- or lactose-intolerant individual who does not have adequate amounts of the enzymes—i.e., maltase and lactase—to digest these foods and obtain their glucose.

- **Intolerance to Dairy Products, Grains or Sugar.**

- **Craving or Thirst for Cold Liquids or Foods.** The person who is carbohydrate deficient is deficient in alkaline minerals, hence too acid (too hot) and desires cold things to cool them down.

- **Sensitivity to Air Pollutants, Such as Perfumes, Smoke, etc.**

- **Poor Tolerance for Stress.** The person who is carbohydrate deficient is already under stress due to a lack of energy. More stress is the straw that breaks the camel's back.

The Enzyme Advantage

- **Strong Desire to Eat Between Meals.** This is the brain demanding the fuel it never got from the meal—glucose.

- **Indigestion, Particularly Two to Three Hours After Eating.**

One of the most puzzling cases I ever encountered involved two women who had come to me from Oklahoma, for environmental allergies—or so they thought.

These were two highly intelligent individuals. One was a medical doctor, the other a paramedical professional. Both had attended my seminars and hoped that I might have a digestive enzyme formula that would help them with their environmental allergies.

Indeed, the particular area of Oklahoma that they were from was home to a large oil refinery complex. And both women realized that when they came to see me, their symptoms went away. It had nothing to do with their diets. "We don't use sugar, and we don't use white flour," the doctor said. "We have perfect diets."

So it made sense that their symptoms were being caused by the environmental toxicants in their home town.

These symptoms included: anxiety, insomnia, inability to handle stress, low energy, headaches, and occasional bowel problems.

People with these symptoms were often put on Librium at the time. They'd been through that, to no avail.

I put them both on a broad digestive enzyme supplement. They were fine, as usual, until they returned to Oklahoma, at which point all their symptoms returned.

Each time they came back, it was the same story. They got better away from home, and when they returned home, they got sick again. None of the enzyme formulas I tried seemed to touch it.

Who could figure it out?

Chapter 4—Carbohydrate: The Perfect Fuel

Finally, I made a trip to Oklahoma to do a seminar, and I told them I wanted to take the two of them to dinner. They asked if they could bring a massage therapist friend along, and I said yes. Charlie sat quietly through the three-hour dinner while I grilled the two women from every possible angle, with no luck.

It all came down to the fact that they ate the healthiest diet, which, at the time, was plenty of vegetables and grains. And they didn't use white sugar or white flour.

"We only eat good," they said.

Finally, Charlie broke in.

"They're lying to you, doc," he said.

"They're what?" I shot back.

He told me that whenever they got frustrated or upset over anything, the two of them would pig out on crackers and bread and stuff like that.

Finally, the ladies 'fessed up, but they insisted that couldn't possibly be the source of their symptoms.

But that was it. I had it. They were both gluten intolerant and experiencing acute hypoglycemia from bingeing out on refined carbohydrates.

And guess what. They didn't bring their crackers and other refined treats with them when they came to visit me.

So it wasn't the air pollution after all.

I ended up going to Anthony Collier and creating a very special formula for them, much like the protease formula that cured my 43-year-long infection in my ears. But this one was a carbohydrate digesting formula heavy in maltase and lactase, as well as invertase, for white sugar. You digest it, the brain is satisfied and doesn't crave it.

It was a charm. Finally, I knew how to diagnose reactive hypoglycemia and what to do for it.

Enough about carbohydrates. Let's see what a protein deficiency looks like.

Chapter 5

Protein: The Body's Second Choice for Energy

It was the biggest discovery of my career, and it was all about protein. Protein and PMS.

Back in the 1960s and 1970s, the medical profession was in the dark when it came to premenstrual syndrome, or "PMS." All they knew was that some women appeared to suffer a wide range of physiological and psychological symptoms during menstruation while others did not. And while the underlying cause of PMS was shrouded in biochemical mystery, if indeed it was biochemically based, the standard course of action was straightforward—just treat the symptoms.

And there were plenty of symptoms to treat. These included everything from bloating, weight gain, fatigue, lack of energy, headaches, cramps, breast swelling and tenderness, to behavioral symptoms, including depression, anger, irritability, aggression, anxiety, decreased alertness, difficulty concentrating, and withdrawal from family and friends.

One study by Columbia University researchers in the 1970s found more than 130 symptoms associated with PMS, which led them to conclude that PMS was not a clinical condition at all. It couldn't be. It just didn't make physiological sense—not with that many symptoms.

A 2012 University of Toronto study came to the same frustrating conclusion. Analyzing 41 research studies tracking women's moods during their menstrual cycles, the researchers were unable to find sufficient evidence that PMS exists.

On the biochemical side, suspected PMS triggers included cyclic changes in hormones and fluctuations of the brain chemical serotonin, which could contribute to depression, fatigue, food cravings and sleep problems.

But that's about it.

The solution: Forget about the cause and just go after the symptoms with drugs. These drugs have included antidepressants, anti-inflammatory drugs (Advil, Motrin, etc.), diuretics to get rid of accumulated fluids that cause the swelling and bloating, and oral contraceptives to shutdown ovulation and stabilize hormonal swings.

Chapter 5—Protein: The Body's Second Choice for Energy

Depo-Provera injections, which are used to stop ovulation in the most severe cases, can actually cause an increase in symptoms, such as increased appetite, weight gain, headache and depression.

So it's a trade-off—side effects for symptom relief.

And yet there is another way.

For the record, PMS is not a "disease," per se. It is not in itself a medical condition, but rather a disruption of normal function, which explains how a health care provider who understands the relationships of anatomy, physiology, neurology and physical diagnosis can find an answer to this health problem using food enzyme nutrition.

This learning curve started for me back in the 1970s, before I began working with enzymes.

Women had been coming to me with PMS from the day I opened my practice. It was a big problem. In an effort to get a handle on the source of their symptoms, I began offering a free 24-hour urinalysis to any PMS patient who would agree to it. What I found was that these women didn't have enough calcium coming out in their urine during menstruation. You're supposed to lose a certain amount of calcium every day. This has been known and documented for well over 100 years. These women were not losing calcium, which told me they were calcium deficient.

It made sense, because calcium is necessary to prevent tetany—muscle spasms or muscle cramps. Furthermore, when a person becomes calcium deficient, they are subject to mood disturbances, such as irritability, anxiety and depression, as well as insomnia—all PMS symptoms. This is due to a related deficiency in serotonin, which is a calming neurotransmitter.

However, the calcium deficiency was not the real culprit. The urine tests also revealed these women were very alkaline, which suggested to me that they were protein deficient, because it's protein that is responsible for buffering excess acidity and alkalinity. And, as noted earlier in this book, protein is responsible for maintaining homeostasis, and this includes the amount of calcium a person has in their blood. Calcium exists in the blood in two forms—free-floating calcium and calcium that is bonded to protein. The ratio of free-floating calcium to calcium bound to protein—approximately 50/50—must never change if homeostasis is to be maintained. As protein levels go down in the blood, so does calcium.

Because homeostasis within the extracellular fluid must be maintained at all costs, the levels of blood protein (albumin) will usually appear normal in these cases. However, due to the energy deficiency, amino acids inside the individual cells are being sent to the liver for conversion to glucose. Hence, the relationship of protein to calcium is disturbed, and the body will lose larger amounts of calcium in the urine until it can no longer afford to do so, at which point lower levels will be excreted. This means the cell is no longer able to respond normally to stimulation from the autonomic nervous system, as discussed in Chapter 4 on carbohydrates.

So while the women I was testing appeared to be calcium deficient, they were in fact protein deficient. That was the cause of their calcium deficiency, as well as their excess alkalinity.

Furthermore, protein attracts water. When a person becomes protein deficient, in addition to calcium, water also leaves the blood. And when water leaves the bloodstream, it collects in the tissues, which results in the edema, or bloating, that women experience during their menstrual cycle.

Chapter 5 — Protein: The Body's Second Choice for Energy

So it all comes down to protein deficiency. The question now became what to do about it? During those first 12 years, I had tried every protein supplement under the sun and I was unable to increase protein use. It wasn't until the early 1980s, after Tony Collier came to my door with Dr. Howell's enzymes, that I was able to put a "dent" in PMS. Because it was a digestion issue—these women simply weren't adequately digesting the protein they were eating.

In my part of the country there was no shortage of protein in the diet. It was a very rural area. We didn't have salad bars. We didn't have vegetarians. Many of the young men were dairy farmers, construction workers, small contractors, etc., who told their wives just what they wanted for dinner—meat, potatoes and gravy. "And don't give me any of that damn rabbit food," pretty much summed it up.

This is still very common in many rural areas today.

So I didn't have to give my female patients protein supplements. What they needed were enzymes to digest the protein they were eating. And that's what I gave them.

I started off with five women who had undergone my 24-hour urinalysis and who had a full range of PMS symptoms. These were all young women with small children. I gave them a multiple food enzyme supplement containing everything they needed to improve digestion, but weighted towards improving protein metabolism.

And I gave them a small amount of calcium—not much, because it's really about protein metabolism.

Their first period after starting the program was the same—no change in symptoms. However, when we checked their urinalysis, we noticed that there was a very definite change in the calcium coming into the urine, as well as a drop in the pH—not quite so alkaline. So I knew I was improving protein digestion.

The big surprise came after their second period. Their symptoms had abated. They were all better—all five of them. It was remarkable.

I had improved protein digestion so they could carry calcium.

This was a huge breakthrough for me in treating women. It is simply not necessary that they should suffer this malady. It's totally unnecessary. *And* it's not natural.

Treating PMS is all about restoring normal function.

The trick is not just treating it when a woman is menstruating, but treating it the entire month. That way, when the body begins to go through its hormonal changes, they will have a normal period without cramping and all the other discomforts.

This plan of action beats going after individual symptoms. If you can restore normal function before a disease can be identified, and then maintain health, you can make a huge difference.

This isn't just about PMS. At least 95 percent of my female patients I treated during the course of my clinical practice were protein deficient at the cellular level.

Once women realize that there is relief from this monthly drudgery, they begin to have hope for other female problems related to protein deficiency that could follow them for the rest of their lives. When a woman's menstrual cycle stops, she experiences hot flashes. We have been able to control hot flashes in thousands of women using protease supplements. It's all about improving protein metabolism and restoring normal function.

Then there's osteoporosis. Bone is made up of protein, calcium and phosphorous. The cause of osteoporosis begins early with a protein

Chapter 5—Protein: The Body's Second Choice for Energy

deficiency and accumulates for years, ending in the chronic degenerative process that is osteoporosis.

Then there's anemia. In my practice, most of the female patients I saw who were anemic were not actually iron-deficient. They were protein deficient.

There are two things a woman needs to metabolize iron to the point where her body is able to use it. First, she needs adequate stomach acid to digest protein. And second, she needs vitamin C, along with the stomach acid, to ionize iron—to turn it from ferric, which the body cannot use, to ferrous, which can be absorbed. The ferrous is then absorbed on a specific protein molecule, called ferritin, and transported on another protein molecule. From there the ferrous is either put into red blood cells in the form of hemoglobin, or it is stored as ferritin on the original protein molecule where it was absorbed.

I have experienced several serendipitous moments with the protein and iron relationship. Back in Chapter 3, we discussed the treatment of the most anemic patient I ever encountered. We also discussed the need for adequate stomach acid and vitamin C (ascorbate) for converting ferric iron to its ferrous form so the body can absorb, transport and use it. And we discussed the spinal innervation of the digestive organs between the shoulder blades. The spleen also sends and receives its communications with the brain from that area, which is in the middle of the large triangular-shaped Trapezius muscle.

Would it come as any surprise that the same herbal/iron-enzyme formula can be used to treat headaches, instead of aspirin, including and especially for children? As a practitioner, I used it on my own children, and I suggested it for my grandchildren.

Speaking of children, do you have a bed wetter in your home? After years of struggling for an answer to that problem, I found a solution when there is no pathology involved. I achieved great success by having the parents reduce the child's sugar intake and improving predigestion with enzymes, and by adding raisins to their daily diet. It takes all three steps to be effective.

I have seen many young women (in their early 30s) who could not get married because they still wet the bed! The cause was the same, with the same three-step solution.

* * *

By definition, proteins, from the Greek word *primary*, are very large naturally occurring molecules, which consist of amino acids made up of carbon, hydrogen, oxygen and nitrogen atoms, as well as sulfur and other elements such as iron and phosphorous.

> **Proteins are essential for all living things, and must therefore be included in the diet to sustain life.**

In nutrition today, great emphasis is placed on consuming a diet that is low in carbohydrates, especially white sugar and flour, in order to prevent weight gain. Great emphasis is also placed on lipids, and what kinds of oils and fatty acids are good for us and which are not—monounsaturated fat, polyunsaturated fat, omega-3 fatty acids, saturated fat, trans fat, and so on.

While all this is important, the *most* important of the three substrates we consume—i.e., protein, carbohydrate and fat—is protein. Protein is the body's sole source of nitrogen. And maintaining a positive nitrogen balance—consuming more protein than one actually needs—is necessary for growth, and life itself.

Chapter 5—Protein: The Body's Second Choice for Energy

When we talk about a young, growing child in a positive nitrogen balance, we are saying that nitrogen is essential for that growth. As we age, we gradually move towards a negative nitrogen balance, where the body does not require as much nitrogen, but a positive nitrogen balance is needed in order to maintain function. Without a positive nitrogen balance, one cannot live.

This being the case, vegetarians can only get nitrogen from vegetables; they cannot get it from fruits. Hence, one cannot become a fruitarian and live.

Again, it comes down to the body's fundamental need for protein. One can avoid meat, but one cannot do without protein.

When it comes to sustaining and keeping the human body in good repair, protein can do almost any of the tasks at hand. In fact, it's almost always involved.

There are two ways of looking at protein's contribution to overall health. One is the functions of dietary proteins; the other is the functions of plasma proteins.

Let's take a look at both.

Dietary Proteins

On the dietary side, there's protein's role in growth and tissue repair, formation of essential body compounds, and antibody formation.

1. **Growth or Increase in Muscle Mass.** This is possible when there is an appropriate mixture of amino acids over and above the amount needed for maintenance (homeostasis) and the

repair of tissue. Some cells require larger amounts of specific amino acids. For example, hair, skin and nails require larger amounts of the sulfur-containing amino acids found in animal protein. Hence, women who struggle with hair, skin and nail problems are usually sulfur deficient, which goes back to protein Sulfur is also needed for cartilage repair.

2. **Formation of Essential Body Compounds.** Whenever there is a protein deficiency, these essential compounds receive priority over other less important protein functions. Hormones such as insulin, epinephrine, and thyroxin are all proteins. Hemoglobin and almost all of the factors involved in blood clotting are also proteins. The photoreceptors in the eye that are responsible for vision are proteins, as are the brain's neurotransmitters dopamine (the alertness chemical) and serotonin (calming chemical).

Once again, homeostasis comes first, followed by the formation of these essential body compounds. Without adequate protein, these essential compounds begin to suffer.

When the body is under stress, it's using a lot of epinephrine (adrenaline). How long can this go on if you're protein deficient?

As noted earlier, it takes eight days for the body to incubate thyroxine. When a person is affected by major stress over an extended period of time, supplies diminish to the point where they need to be put on Synthroid.

Then there's serotonin—the alertness chemical.

All of these essential compounds suffer in times of protein deficiency.

3. **Finally, There's Antibody Formation.** Protein deficiency accounts for a large amount of infant mortality among malnourished children because specific antibodies against

infection cannot be formed. And if a woman is protein deficient when she becomes pregnant, she is probably going to be protein deficient throughout the pregnancy, as the demands of the baby have to be met.

Taking in the bigger picture, one has only to think how many chronic immune problems there are in the world today that modern research continues to explore.

Plasma Proteins

The proteins that reside in the blood, the plasma proteins, are responsible for maintaining homeostasis. They are not used by cells to facilitate energy production, growth or repair. Plasma proteins are made in the liver; their sole purpose is to maintain homeostasis.

For plasma proteins, these tasks include: the maintenance of acid-alkaline balance (pH), regulation of water balance, transport of nutrients and waste, and the removal of toxic compounds.

Looking at each of these functions, we learn that:

1. **Acid/Alkaline Balance.** The body's effort to maintain an acid/alkaline balance is a behind-the-scenes struggle that goes on 24/7 without us even being aware of it. Plasma proteins are buffers that have the ability to neutralize excess acid and alkali in the blood, thus maintaining a normal acid-base balance. The blood has to be maintained within a certain narrow limit of pH. Any deviation can mean a trip to the emergency room.

2. **Regulation of Water Balance.** Plasma proteins are like magnets. They attract water and hold it in solution. Water moves towards protein. It's that simple. Just as protein holds

water inside the shock-absorbing vertebral discs, plasma protein molecules pull fluid from between the cells back into the bloodstream, maintaining the critical "osmotic" balance that is key to maintaining homeostasis. The accumulation of fluid in the tissues is an early warning sign of protein deficiency. Excess fluid gives tissues a soft, spongy, bloated appearance, as in the case of a protein deficiency and bloating that comes with menstruation.

The maintenance of water balance in the body is critical.

In 2007, a 28-year-old California woman died after taking part in a drinking contest held by a radio station in which the person who drank the most water would win a car. This woman drank so much water that her extracellular fluids became diluted and excessively low in sodium and other electrolytes, compared to the fluids inside her body cells. As a result, extracellular water began forcing its way into the woman's cells, to balance the concentration. This caused her brain to swell up, and she died.

Extremes aside, it's protein that maintains the delicate day-to-day extracellular and intracellular water balance in our bodies.

3. **Transport of Nutrients and Waste.** In a word, proteins play an essential role in the transport of nutrients across the intestinal wall into the blood, from the blood to the tissues, and across the cell membranes into the cell. Most of the transportation of nutrients to the cells and waste from the cells to the kidneys and lungs is done by plasma proteins:

- Calcium is carried by protein.

- Iron is carried by protein.

- Cholesterol is carried by protein.

- Hormones are carried by protein.

Chapter 5—Protein: The Body's Second Choice for Energy

You name it, protein carries it.

And so it follows, when there is an inadequate supply of protein, less of these carrier proteins are available, and the transportation of nutrients and the removal of cellular waste products can become impaired, and with it, homeostasis.

4. The Role of Proteins in the Removal of Toxic Compounds.
For plasma proteins, this task involves attaching to the toxic substances and transporting them to the kidney, which is the great arbitrator. It's up to the kidney to sort out what to keep in the body and what to discard. As for the detoxification process itself, this is performed primarily by enzymes—aka proteins—found in the liver.

Again, one would be hard pressed to find anything taking place in the body that does not involve the conspicuously oversized, all-important protein molecule.

Now let's take a look at what a protein deficiency looks like.

Protein Deficiency Has Many Faces

I am often asked, "How much protein should I be eating?"

It is impossible to answer this question without knowing how much protein your body needs to meet its energy demands, which depends on your lifestyle; how much protein you are currently consuming; and finally, how much you are actually digesting and absorbing.

How much protein does your body need?

We've talked about the many functions of protein and how important it is, in terms of maintaining homeostasis and keeping our body cells in good repair. Proteins are the primary nutrient for maintaining normal body functions. So it should come as no surprise that each individual's brain is accustomed to receiving a certain amount of protein on a regular basis. In other words, each of us consumes about the same amount of protein every day.

If we do not consume adequate amounts of protein or adequately digest the protein we consume, we will crave sweets as the body cries out for that quick energy fix.

So how much protein does your body require? The generally accepted daily dietary allowance is 0.8 grams of protein per kilogram of bodyweight. This can be found in any nutritional textbook. Loosely translated, it means that you need approximately 3.2 grams per 10 pounds of bodyweight to maintain your present weight.

However, there are no average people! That figure is used for a sedentary lifestyle and there are many other variables that come into play with each individual.

Age, for instance. Young individuals need more protein for growth. Bone formation is not complete until age 20, or thereabouts. Older people need to reduce their calories, but not protein.

What is your lifestyle? Do you lead a fairly sedentary life, with light exercise, such as regular walking, or do you have a more extensive workout routine?

How much stress do you encounter during the day? This is a widely misunderstood concept. Again, we're not just talking about mental stress. It can be structural stress, relating to an individual's daily struggle to remain upright in a world governed by the force of gravity, or it can refer to visceral or emotional stresses, all of which can require more nutrition. So do you drive a beer truck? Do you

Chapter 5—Protein: The Body's Second Choice for Energy

spend your days hauling heavy cases of beer in and out of stores all day long? Or are you a stay at home mom, or an empty nester?

A tournament chess player, perhaps?

Or are you a vegetarian? Please know that plant proteins are incomplete proteins, in the sense that they don't contain all of the essential amino acids—the amino acids our bodies require but do not have the ability to synthesize. The nine amino acids we humans cannot synthesize are: phenylalanine, valine, threonine, tryptophan, methionine, leucine, isoleucine, lysine, and histidine. We must get these from foods we eat.

True vegetarians must be very careful to mix and match the vegetables they eat to get all the different types of amino acids needed to maintain health. It can be done, but you really have to know what you are doing to get a balanced amino acid picture, using combinations of foods, such as corn and beans, soybeans and rice, or red beans, which are a better source of essential amino acids.

Some vegetarians become "ovotarians," incorporating eggs, which are by far the best source of protein on the planet.

> **Many young women I have encountered during the course of my practice consider themselves to be vegetarians when in reality they are what I call "pasta-tarians." They're eating pasta to avoid meat. For the record, neither white rice or wild rice, or pasta are good sources of essential amino acids.**

Further, the way the body uses amino acids is not helter-skelter, but rather, a very delicate orchestration, making supplementation a rather complicated affair.

> ## Food *for* Thought
>
> **Further, think of the hypothalamus as the conductor of an amino acid orchestra consisting of 30 violins, 12 cellos, 10 double basses, an assortment of woodwind instruments, four flutes, four oboes, four clarinets, four bassoons, eight French horns, six trumpets, six trombones, one tuba, a piano, and a full percussion section, with one lone musician alternating between cymbals and the triangle.**

Back in the 1970s, they were going to transform medicine by using individual amino acids, but it didn't work. Why? Because the hypothalamus said "I don't need any more violins. I don't care how good he is, I don't need him."

Again, 95 percent of my female patients have turned out to be protein deficient. Most of the health care practitioners who I have examined personally, who are on raw food diets, or vegan diets, because they believe philosophically that it is the healthiest way to go, are protein deficient. This is true of the best of them.

A person is not going to know they are protein deficient until they develop symptoms. Blood tests are not the answer. Because the body's number one priority is always to maintain homeostasis. The blood tests hospitals use to measure the amount of protein in the blood will always come up normal, until you're really sick. A protein-deficiency diagnosis can be determined with blood tests, but only if one looks at

Chapter 5—Protein: The Body's Second Choice for Energy

the homeostatic relationship between protein, calcium and phosphorus.

Or the diagnosis can be made with a 24-hour urine sample and a hands-on examination by a health care provider who is trained in uncovering nutritional deficiencies by tracking involuntary muscle contractions to their visceral source (or sources). It can be a complicated process, in some cases involving multiple nutritional deficiencies and multiple organ systems.

One of the most surprising cases I ever encountered involved a middle-aged woman who came to my office with lingering pain in the small of her back due to an injury she suffered when she fell off her chair at work. After months of suffering despite treatment from several sources, she turned to chiropractic.

It was the early 1980s. I had just started using food enzymes with protein supplements to treat people with intervertebral disc problems. Improvement in such cases was slow, but I was able to provide significant relief, which encouraged patients to stay the course.

Examination of this woman failed to reveal a structural problem—her disc was not deflated. Rather, the area around the disc had been injured, and the annulus, the rubber band-like ligaments that hold the disc in place and keep it under pressure, was stretched out and not healing. In injury cases such as this, the water inside the disc is not under adequate pressure, which can cause problems. However, this woman had not reached the point where we could demonstrate on an X-ray that she had a deflated disc. At this point, it was all about restoring the integrity of the annulus.

The major component of the annulus is vitamin C. If the annulus is vitamin C deficient, it will begin to stretch. She wasn't really protein deficient. She was vitamin C deficient. So I gave her a formula

I had developed that contained protein and vitamin C, and enzymes to digest the protein. I told her I thought that this might strengthen the area where she was having her pain, and that she should go home and take two capsules every four hours, and then three capsules with each meal starting the next day.

I adjusted her back, which helped relieve some of the muscle contraction problems, but I knew that wouldn't last. I had no idea how long it was going to take for her body to heal. I was completely blown away when she called me at 7 o'clock that night and told me that her pain was completely gone!

"Are you sure?" I said.

"Yes," she said. "This is unbelievable!"

She asked me if she should keep taking them, and I said to do just as I had told her.

Three or four days later, she came to see me, and she was fine. I just left her taking the formula with every meal for a while and she never had pain again.

But the way it happened—so fast! She'd been in continuous pain for months.

For the first time I saw that by using enzymes to predigest the nutrients, I could bypass an incompetent digestive system and deliver nutrients into the blood right out of the stomach. I could deliver the necessary nutrition and relieve muscle contractions in just 30 minutes!

That's what I was doing with her.

If the ligaments that hold your joints together are not strong, not as strong as they *should be* because they have been injured and stretched, then the muscles around the spine have to try to hold it together. These muscles fatigue very quickly. And because they're using nutrition in huge amounts, they become energy deficient.

Chapter 5—Protein: The Body's Second Choice for Energy

When you start pumping much-needed nutrients into the body, these muscles are suddenly getting all the nutrition they need and they are strong again in 30 minutes.

And that's how this formula worked for her.

After that, all I had to do as a chiropractor was keep her back aligned while the ligaments shrunk. It took 60 to 90 days of vitamin C delivery for the ligaments that make up the annulus to regain their integrity. Thus, we prevented chronic degeneration in that area.

Basically, she needed protein to give her muscles the energy they required to handle the extra work, and vitamin C for ligament repair.

One could say she was not protein deficient, and yet she was.

* * *

So what are the warning signs of protein deficiency? What symptoms suggest that you are not consuming or digesting adequate amounts of protein to meet your body needs?

- **You Crave Sweets.** Again, when you run low on carbohydrates for energy, your body turns to protein for conversion into glucose. That is why people under chronic stress are protein deficient. You might think the body would crave high protein foods, but no, it wants the "quicker fix." It's not going for the hamburger, it's going for the bun. Better yet, it wants sugar, and it wants it now!

- **Fatigue.** This is the most common complaint voiced by patients entering doctors' offices. Fatigue has many causes, one of which can be protein deficiency. It's all about energy. Your body is struggling to maintain homeostasis in the midst of ongoing structural, visceral and emotional challenges, and you don't have enough protein for energy. And let's not forget iron. You've got to have protein to transport iron, and to absorb it, or you're going to become anemic.

- **Swelling of the Hands and Feet.** Edema, or water gain, which appears as a collection of fluid under the skin, most commonly affects the legs, feet, and ankles. As we've seen in women with PMS, one of the important functions of protein is to maintain water in the blood. Protein is a magnet for water. When you are protein deficient, water will leave the blood and collect in the tissues. Another tell-tale sign of a protein deficiency is increased water secretions coming from your mouth, nose or eyes. Again, protein is the magnet, and when you're deficient, you can lose water. It's that simple.

- **Cold Hands and Feet.** This again is related to protein holding water in the blood. As water is lost, the warming effect that full blood circulation provides is reduced.

- **Muscle Tension Headache.** I have found that in many cases, these chronic, recurring headaches can involve a digestive problem caused by an energy deficiency when carbohydrates are used up and the body starts converting protein for energy. The organs of digestion are enervated in the middle of the thoracic spine, between the shoulder blades. Imagine an inverted pyramid. A muscle, the trapezius, runs from the spine in the area of the kidneys upward and over the shoulder blades, to the outward points of the shoulders, and then up to the base of the skull. If there is any visceral dysfunction, involving the kidney, digestive, or other organs that share innervation with this muscle, the resulting involuntary muscle contraction pulling on the base of the skull will eventually produce a headache.

- **Skin Rashes.** Most skin rashes, which may or may not be accompanied by dry or flaking skin, can be a symptom of a protein deficiency. More involved rashes, such as dermatitis, eczema, and psoriasis, have more complicated issues and will be discussed in the next chapter.

More complicated issues are inevitable with protein-related symptoms. This stems from the fact that protein has important homeostatic relationships with other nutrients, such as calcium, sulfur, magnesium, phosphorus, iron, cholesterol, vitamin C and the entire vitamin B complex.

Consider the following:

- **Anxiety, Irritability, Restlessness.** As discussed earlier in this chapter, anxiety and restlessness are associated with the protein-calcium bond, with a deficiency in protein leading to a deficiency in blood-borne calcium. This relationship also accounts for muscle cramps, menstrual cramps, and difficulty tolerating exercise, which is frequently related to the following:

- **Stiff, Sore Joints.** Protein, calcium and phosphorous have relationships with each other. There's a balance between protein and calcium, and a balance between calcium and phosphorous. All three make up bone. If you are deficient in any of these, protein being the key, you've got stiff, sore joints. Do you have frequent writer's cramp, or are you a slow morning starter? This is most often associated with the protein and phosphorus relationship.

- **Thinning or Brittle Hair.** Hair is made up of protein and specific amino acids that contain sulfur. Hence, a deficiency may lead to your hair lacking the amount of sulfur it needs to stay healthy.

- **Ridges in Fingernails.** Sulfur is also needed in the fingernails. Furthermore, white lines or spots in the fingernails and toenails can be caused by a lack of protein and zinc in the diet. Zinc is involved in 40 different metabolic enzymes in the human body. According to experts, the entire human race is borderline zinc deficient.

- **Difficulty Sleeping.** This can be caused by a serotonin deficiency, which in turn can be caused by a lack of the amino acid tryptophan. The absence of serotonin is often responsible for the inability to relax, to become serene, and to drift off to sleep easily. The lack of specific minerals like potassium and magnesium may also result in the inability to sleep.

- **Slow Healing.** Patients who do not heal or rebound quickly after an illness or injury are often protein deficient. The body needs protein to repair tissue. Amino acids, the building blocks of protein, are crucial to this process.

- **Unexplained Weight Loss.** This always involves protein. In the case of muscle wasting, the body is actually breaking down muscle tissue to get at protein. It may indicate something very serious requiring immediate medical attention, such as a cancer that is using the body's protein to facilitate it's own exponential growth.

The signs and symptoms of protein deficiency are indeed many and varied, with a lot of overlap when it comes to related deficiencies of essential vitamins and minerals. This made for some very tricky trial-and-error diagnoses on my own part, as I pursued this winding learning curve.

Chapter 5—Protein: The Body's Second Choice for Energy

About Hot Flashes

One particularly challenging case involved a middle-aged woman suffering from severe hot flashes. She had been everywhere and tried everything with no luck. When she came to me, back in 1985, she was desperate. She was actually running the air-conditioner in her car in January!

So where does one start? I was having success with protein and calcium supplements with enzymes for PMS, but this was an entirely different ball game. This was my first case of hot flashes. I mean, how many women come to a chiropractor for hot flashes?

I examined her, ran the usual blood and urine tests, and found that she was protein deficient. Just like the PMS patients. So I started her out on the same regimen, with doses of food enzymes to improve predigestion of the protein supplements I was giving her, along with small inclusions of calcium and vitamin C.

It didn't touch it. It worked for PMS, but not for hot flashes. There was no change in the severity or frequency of this woman's hot flashes, and, oddly enough, no change in her lab results!

I had never seen that before—improved digestion and utilization of protein without any substantial change in examination findings. No effect whatsoever.

It's easy to dismiss the problem as being hormonal, and yes, there were examination findings of hormonal imbalance. But she was being treated medically for that, and I wasn't about to interfere with those treatments. I was out to improve nutrition. Period.

Now it also turned out that this woman had a history of heartburn, or acid indigestion, which got me thinking about how hormones need lipids. Then it finally dawned on me. Okay, I thought. She's protein deficient, which means she's hydrochloric acid deficient, and hydrochloric acid stimulates the flow of bile. So she's not digesting fat very well either. If I can improve her ability to digest fat as well as protein, that should improve her hormone imbalance.

Well, we gave her heavy lipase supplementation and the lipid situation straightened out. She was digesting fat. And we continued with the protein protocol, so she was digesting plenty of protein. But still no luck. Her examination findings were improving, but there was no change in her hot flashes. Her symptoms weren't improving.

Finally, I began to think maybe it was the mix of amino acids. As noted earlier, plant proteins do not have a complete complement of amino acids. So I put her on an improved protein supplement—egg protein, which has a fully balanced amount of amino acids.

I was giving her better protein, she was digesting the protein, and she should have been getting better, but she still wasn't quite there.

That's when I figured it out. I knew it had to be the amino acids. Maybe I just didn't have enough violins. It turned out I needed another cello player, and that cellist was sulfur. So I simply bumped in some amino acids that contained sulfur, and that did the trick. It took a while, but her hot flashes went away.

I know eggs contain sulfur, but in this case not enough to overcome her deficiency fast enough—fast enough being the optimal phrase.

> **I finally had the fix for hot flashes. But it's not the same for every patient. Every patient is different. There are no magic bullets. You give the body the specific nutrition it needs and then wait for it to heal itself. That was the secret to getting rid of hot flashes.**

Chapter 5—Protein: The Body's Second Choice for Energy

That's the way it is with any protein deficiency. When it comes to body chemistry and maintaining homeostasis, protein is connected to everything.

Now let's move on to fats.

Chapter 6

Lipid: The Last Resort

One of the most rewarding cases ever to come my way was a woman—a physician—who had failed to become pregnant despite four years of trying everything under the sun.

She'd been through it all.

After a year of trying to conceive naturally, she and her husband were both medically evaluated. The first course of action was the surgical treatment of her husband to remove a varicocele (an abnormal enlargement of the venous plexus in the scrotum) and a spermatocele (a retention cyst of the tubule in the testes).

After months of waiting and still no pregnancy, the couple tried intrauterine injection (IUI), which involves artificial insemination of the sperm into the uterus.

Again, no luck.

The next step to consider was in vitro fertilization (IVF), which involves close monitoring and stimulating of the woman's ovulatory process, removing the ovum, or eggs, from the ovaries, and exposing them to sperm in a fluid medium in the laboratory. After that, the fertilized egg is cultured for two to six days in a growth medium and then implanted in the woman's uterus.

But why should she go through with such a "scary" procedure, when the doctors reviewing all of her tests kept saying that they could find nothing wrong with her?

Why do it? It made no sense.

So continued searching. She tried various holistic treatments, like acupuncture, chiropractic, herbs, homeopathy, naturopathy, yoga therapy to reduce stress—she was going through a particularly challenging time in her life—along with various supplements and dietary changes, and a heap of prayer.

Again, no luck. She just couldn't conceive.

By the time she came to me, my job was easier because she was already working on stress reduction, which was contributing to her inability to conceive, in that stress, as we have seen, contributes to nutritional deficiencies.

So we began taking the steps dictated by her body.

We started out making specific structural corrections, with specific nutritional support to heal the tissues involved.

Second came dietary changes. It was a very complicated case. Fortunately I had a very compliant patient.

Third, digestion had to be improved via enzyme supplementation, in order to improve stomach and biliary functions.

Finally, we were able to begin to nourish her with formulas

Chapter 6—Lipid: The Last Resort

designed to normalize lipid metabolism, and thus energize the hormonal system.

Mother Nature did the rest.

The bottom line: It's amazing what the human body can do when it functions normally. The final nutritional adjustments were made in January and she was pregnant in February. She gave birth to a healthy baby boy in November. Her second son was born eighteen months later. Every so often I get pictures of two of the best-looking healthy boys you can imagine.

* * *

Isn't it interesting that all the hormonal organs—the pituitary gland, the thyroid, and both the adrenal medulla and the adrenal cortex—respond to the "fight or flight" stress response calling, but not the reproductive hormone-producing organs. This is because the lipids—aka fats—these organs need to make reproduction possible are being used for energy! And yet, no creature on Earth could be conceived without them.

That's right, reproductive problems, along with various hormonal issues, both male and female, may in fact be related to inadequate lipid ingestion and/or inadequate lipid digestion, because when push comes to shove, the hypothalamus considers the energy production needed to sustain life—i.e., maintain homeostasis—to be more important than reproduction.

How long is this supposed to go on? It's one thing to divert lipid energy from the reproductive organs in an acute or temporary situation; it's quite another to divert it in a chronic or lifestyle situation.

Lipid metabolism is fundamental to life itself, and to the maintenance of good health. And yet, in spite of all the attention lipids receive, or because of all the misinformation generated by product advertising hype, dietary fats—i.e., saturated fat, unsaturated fat, trans fat, monounsaturated fat, polyunsaturated fat, omega-3 fatty acids, omega-6s, good fats, bad fats, you name it—are a source of much confusion in the minds of the general public.

But this misinformation need not be the case.

Let's start at the top this time. What does a lipid deficiency look like?

Symptoms Of A Lipid Deficiency

First, a lipid deficiency, like a carbohydrate or protein deficiency, can result from inadequate ingestion of healthy fatty acids or the inability to digest fats.

Second, the more common symptoms that occur as one progresses from a carbohydrate deficiency, where you lose water and become dry, to a protein deficiency, where you develop edema in your hands and feet, along with skin, hair and nail problems, can all be found in a lipid deficiency in varying degrees from individual to individual, along with vision, sleep and mood disorders. The symptoms can accumulate as one progresses from one deficiency to the next, and the picture becomes more and more complicated.

When I was in practice, patients would occasionally call in saying they had to cancel their appointment that day because they had the flu.

"I can't come in today," they would say, "because I have bone-aching flu. I hurt all over and I'm running a temperature. I can't even get out of bed."

"If you can make it," my assistant would respond, "come in your pajamas and your bathrobe. I'll meet you at the back door and take you in the back treatment room. Chances are, in an hour and a half,

Chapter 6—Lipid: The Last Resort

you'll go home and you won't have any more fever and you won't hurt."

The words "bone-aching" were the tip-off. When they said bone aching, I was pretty sure it was about fat and not the flu.

When the patient arrived, I would palpate them. In this case, the universal stress point is up in the shoulders. When that continues long enough, the stress points for reproduction, which are halfway between your belly button and the pubic area, become positive with involuntary muscle contractions. You can palpate those contractions and that confirms that the patient is fat deficient. They're under stress, they've gone through their stored energy supplies of carbohydrate and protein, and now they're using up their stored fats, to the point where the endocrine system has become overtaxed and it's unable to produce enough of the steroid hormone cortisol.

That's where the bone pain comes from. Low cortisol, the stress hormone, results in bone pain.

So what appears to be the flu is actually a cascade of symptoms resulting from an energy deficiency as the body goes through its stored supplies of carbohydrate, protein, and now lipids.

After making the specific, indicated spinal adjustments, I would treat these patients with one of two formulas I had developed for male and female reproductive issues. These consist of lipid, protein and carbohydrate herbal supplements (lipid-rich saw palmetto, and other herbs), and the lipase, protease and amylase enzymes they needed to digest these herbs.

I'd give the patients four capsules, cover them with a quilt, and 45 minutes later I'd come back to the treatment room, palpate them again for the muscle contractions, and adjust the vertebrae again. Then I'd give them four more capsules, and 45 minutes later, all their symptoms—fever, bone pain, all of it!—would be gone and they'd want to go home.

> **In such cases, give the body the nutrition it needs, and the symptoms will disappear, as opposed to just going after the symptoms with drugs, which would have been marginally palliative at best. It is all part of the sympathetic cascade as the patients progress from carbohydrate to protein and finally to lipid deficiency.**

Again, the bone-aching was the tip-off—and the involuntary muscle contractions on examination that pointed to the hormone deficiency that pointed to the lipid deficiency.

The most devastating symptoms occur when the body's stores of carbohydrate and protein run low, and are forced to turn to lipids for energy. Lipids would otherwise be used to produce reproductive hormones and other essential compounds.

For example, when the body is forced to pull stored fats into the blood for conversion to glucose for energy, it must also slow down insulin production. Otherwise, the insulin would be used to move the glucose into all the body's cells, when it (mostly) needs to be saved for use by the brain, and a little for the reproductive system.

Finally, because most lipids are not water soluble—rather than being taken up directly to the liver as proteins and carbohydrates are—they must be absorbed into the lymphatic system and pumped

Chapter 6—Lipid: The Last Resort

around the body and then finally to the liver. That's right. Lipids play an important role in the immune system too.

Let's back up now, and take a closer look at the role lipids play in the body, and see what a lipid deficiency looks like *from the inside out*, as the body works to absorb these key nutrients. It's a fascinating glimpse at the genius of Nature that went into the design of the human body.

Then we'll cut through all the hype and look at which of the many available over-the-counter alternatives are most likely to relieve the symptoms of a lipid deficiency.

> **Food *for* Thought**
>
> **I have already expressed my opinion that there are no "magic bullets" in nutrition.**

Lipids are essential dietary ingredients. The body is capable of synthesizing lipids, or fatty acids, from protein and carbohydrate, except for three "essential fatty acids," which the body must, therefore, obtain from foods. These essential fatty acids include: linoleic, linolenic and arachidonic acid.

Linoleic acid is a polyunsaturated omega-6 fatty acid found in vegetable and seed oils. Linolenic acid is a polyunsaturated omega-3 fatty acid found in plants, seeds, nuts, many common vegetable oils, and fish, such as salmon and mackerel. Arachidonic acid can be converted from linoleic acid, and is, therefore, not absolutely essential. It is found in animal fat.

These essential fatty acids are known to improve dermatitis and have been shown to restore growth to young animals fed a fat-deficient diet. For example, essential fatty acid deficiencies are most commonly found in babies fed a nonfat formula. Males need more essential fatty acids than females, but females have more difficulty digesting fats.

So what happens to fatty acids when they are finally broken down for use by the body? They wind up as leukotrienes, thromboxanes and prostaglandins, all of which are hormone-like lipid compounds that act as local messenger molecules.

Leukotrienes were first discovered in white blood cells (leukocytes), which is how they got their name, though they have since been found in other immune cells. Leukotrienes help regulate immune responses and are usually accompanied by the production of histamine and prostaglandins, which also act to regulate inflammation. So if you are leukotriene-deficient, you are probably under medical care.

Thromboxanes are named for their role in clot formation (thrombosis). In other words, they facilitate the clumping together of blood platelets. They also constrict blood vessels and thereby raise blood pressure locally. Again, if you have problems here, you are likely to be under medical care.

Prostaglandins are also derived from fatty acids and have very important functions in the body. These hormone-like substances regulate the contraction and relaxation of smooth muscles—the muscles that humans cannot control voluntarily. Prostaglandins are found within the walls of blood vessels, lymphatic vessels, gastrointestinal tract, respiratory tract, and the urinary bladder, even the male and female reproductive tracts. They also promote conception, induce labor, and regulate transmission of nerve signals.

Chapter 6—Lipid: The Last Resort

The name "prostaglandins" dates back to a time when they were first observed in the seminal fluid and were believed to be secreted by the prostate gland. It was later shown, however, that they are produced by the seminal vesicles, and that many other tissues secrete prostaglandins.

Prostaglandins act on different receptor sites to influence an array of physiological effects in addition to those mentioned above. Among their many functions, prostaglandins:

- Act on specialized cells in the kidney to increase its rate of filtration.
- Regulate calcium movement.
- Regulate hormones.
- Act on cells in the stomach wall to inhibit acid secretion.
- Decrease intraocular pressure within the eye—i.e., glaucoma.
- Sensitize the spinal nerves to pain.
- Regulate the inflammatory response by the white blood cells.
- Cause ion aggregation or disaggregation of platelets—i.e., blood clotting.

It's now known that aspirin-like drugs inhibit the synthesis of prostaglandins.

How critical are prostaglandins? Suffice it to say that when you're deficient in prostaglandins, you cannot reproduce.

A woman can't get pregnant. If she gets pregnant, she cannot stay pregnant. If she does carry to term, she cannot induce labor by herself. And even if her baby is delivered by cesarean, she cannot lactate adequately to feed her baby.

**Prostaglandins are the jewels
at the end of the fat chain.**

And recognizing a prostaglandin deficiency is the starting point in making a diagnosis. From there you backpedal. You analyze it back to the patient's diet. Is it that they are not digesting what they are eating? Or, is it that they're not eating it? Are they eating the wrong kinds of foods? Are they using oils, which are coating their foods and making them more difficult to digest? Or, are they under so much stress that they're burning up their fats?

Why are they deficient in prostaglandins? That's the question that needs to be answered.

* * *

Now let's talk about how your body takes in foods that contain fatty acids, and slowly and methodically turns them into the aforementioned molecules, prostaglandins being the principal, and most important, end product we should be most interested in.

We begin by looking at what might be regarded as the Rodney Dangerfield of the modern diet—enzymes, in particular food enzymes. Why Rodney Dangerfield? Because while they are vital in the digestive-absorption sequence of fat metabolism, as the endearingly self-deprecating comedian said, "They get no respect." Enzymes are widely misunderstood and unappreciated.

The first thing one needs to realize is that enzymes cannot penetrate oils. However, they can digest fats in foods, such as bananas and olives.

With that in mind, let's start in the mouth.

Chapter 6—Lipid: The Last Resort

Lipase Activity In The Mouth

This is where it all starts.

The body places enzymes in its saliva. To get lipid digestion started, a weak lipase is secreted from under the tongue when food is chewed. While the food is not in the mouth long enough for digestion to occur, this enzyme, like the food enzymes, works in the pH range of the resting stomach, alongside supplemental food enzyme lipase, before stomach acid is produced. What is remarkable about sublingual and gastric lipase is the fact that they have the ability to work without the aid of emulsifying bile salts.

But sublingual and gastric lipase only begin to digest long-chain triglycerides (fat-soluble triglycerides) into partial glycerides and free fatty acids. Nevertheless, as much as 30 percent of fat can be digested this way within one to 20 minutes of ingestion by sublingual lipase alone! Recall that it will take the body at least 45 minutes on average to make stomach acid.

Digestion of dietary fats is essential for fat absorption by the small intestine, since long-chain fatty acids, which include the previously mentioned essential fatty acids, cannot be taken directly to the liver for detoxification. Instead, they must be absorbed into the lymphatic system and eventually pumped into the blood, taken through the heart, and finally to the liver.

Is your oil supplement composed of long-chain fatty acids? Probably. Again, enzymes can't penetrate oil.

This is the problem with oil supplements. If you're a health care provider with a patient who is fatty acid deficient, vitamin A deficient, vitamin D deficient, vitamin E deficient (all fat-soluble vitamins), you can't give them oil supplements with their meals, because they've already proven they cannot digest oil. This is just going to coat their meal with oil and make their problem worse. If you want to use oil supplements, it's best to give them to the patient on an empty stomach—i.e., between meals—with the hope that some of it will be absorbed.

Lipase Activity In The Stomach

Moving down into the stomach, a gastric lipase is secreted by gastric chief cells (aka peptic cells, gastric zymogenic cells)—the same cells that secrete pepsinogen to be converted into pepsin for protein digestion.

Gastric lipase works in an acid pH range of 3 to 6. Like sublingual lipase, gastric lipase does not require bile to emulsify fats, as do the lipases that will be secreted by the pancreas into the duodenum. The gastric lipase performs most of the work itself, and in newborns this enzyme provides up to 50 percent of the total breakdown of fats.

As important as they are in the digestion and absorption of dietary fats, sublingual and gastric lipases have a significant limitation; they only remove one fatty acid from each triglyceride molecule. That fatty acid can cross the epithelial membrane lining the intestine and enter the body. But the other two fatty acids are still connected to the glycerol molecule and they cannot enter the body yet.

Not yet.

This is where the action of bile comes in—to break down these two remaining fatty acids in the duodenum. Nevertheless, the action of the sublingual and gastric lipases, along with food enzyme lipase, are critical because the presence of the monoglycerides and diglycerides they create work to improve the action of bile.

Chapter 6—Lipid: The Last Resort

> **Food *for* Thought**
>
> **Howell had it right.**
> **Sooner or later, it all comes back to the worker enzymes.**

Bile—Your Body's Degreaser

All of this said, if there is one stand-out player in this finely tuned orchestration of lipid metabolism, that player would have to be bile. It's the bile that breaks fats into small enough particles with enough surface area for the lipase to penetrate their bonds and break them up for digestion and absorption.

> **Bile is the Dawn dishwashing liquid of the digestive system without which fat absorption could not take place. Period.**

Try washing greasy dishes without Dawn, or some such product.

Bile is particularly critical when it comes to breaking down oils, which do not contain food enzymes, and which neither supplemental enzymes nor the body's own lipase can penetrate.

Bile is alkaline and can help neutralize stomach acid as it enters the duodenum, or small intestine. This is important because pancreatic lipase requires an alkaline environment to be active. This also points to the important fact that it is the presence of stomach acid that stimulates the flow of bile, not the presence of dietary fat.

Some foods, such as cucumbers, onions, radishes and cabbage, including sauerkraut, contain chemicals that also stimulate the flow of bile. This is why I always removed these foods from a patient's diet, along with fried foods and pork, if I was treating them for biliary dysfunction.

More to the point is that we are a population who now buys in the neighborhood of $3 billion of over-the-counter protein pump inhibitors annually for the treatment of gastroesophageal reflux "disease"—aka GERD, acid reflux disease, or gastritis. The idea is to knock out stomach acid production to relieve the symptoms. Unfortunately, this also retards the flow of bile and its ability to do its job.

Furthermore, while it's called gastroesophageal reflux disease, it is not actually a disease; it's a disorder. Again, the pharmacologic approach is all about treating symptoms and not the underlying deficiency that is culminating in the symptoms. Proton pump inhibitors are routinely "thrown at" any symptoms of digestive disorder, often with no examination. When used appropriately, short-term, these drugs can be helpful, to give the mucosal lining of the esophagus a break and time to heal. Too often, however, people wind up taking them long-term, sometimes for years. With stomach acid reduced, protein digestion is also reduced in the stomach, as well as the flow of bile, which reduces lipid digestion.

Good bile flow is critical to good lipid digestion. Many do not realize that bile is produced continuously by the liver and drips into the gallbladder, which is nothing more than a purse, storing the bile until it is prompted by hormonal messengers to squeeze out its contents as food passes out of the stomach and into the small intestine.

If, on the other hand, there is little need for bile to provide alkalinity and water to the small intestine, due to an absence of stomach acid, the bile becomes thick and doesn't flow as readily as it should. Its water content is actually reabsorbed back into the body. This makes for a sluggish bile, which, besides impairing fat and fat-soluble vitamin absorption (vitamins A, D, E and K), can result in gallstone formation, eventually necessitating the removal of the gallbladder.

After the gallbladder is removed, the consistency of the bile doesn't change. The restriction to the flow of bile (the stones) has been removed, but the symptoms often return within two to three years.

In other words, it isn't the gallbladder that is at fault after all—it's the diet and lack of stomach acid! And the long-term use of proton pump inhibitors, which is short-sighted, at best.

In summary, bile salts secreted by the liver and stored in the gallbladder are released into the small intestine, where they coat and emulsify large fat droplets into smaller droplets, thus exposing increased surface area, which makes it possible for the pancreatic lipase to break apart the fat more effectively. Pancreatic lipase is the primary enzyme that breaks down dietary fat, converting the triglycerides found in ingested oils (once they are emulsified) to monoglycerides and free fatty acids.

The bottom line: Without bile, nothing flows.

LIPID ABSORPTION

Here's where the real magic begins.

Bile contains water and bile salts, and some minerals. Bile molecules are two-sided. On one side, they are hydrophilic (water-loving), and on the other side they are hydrophobic (water-hating). Thus, bile molecules tend to aggregate around droplets of lipids (triglycerides and phospholipids) to form micelles, an aggregate of molecules, with their hydrophobic sides facing towards the fat, and their hydrophilic sides facing outwards.

The hydrophilic sides are negatively charged. This negative charge prevents the fat droplets coated with bile from re-aggregating into larger fat particles.

The dispersion of food fat into micelles thus provides a greatly increased surface area so the pancreatic lipase is now able to reach the fatty core through gaps between the bile salts, and digest the triglycerides.

The pancreatic lipase breaks down each triglyceride into two fatty acids and a monoglyceride, which are then absorbed by the villi on the intestine walls. After being transferred across the intestinal membrane, the fatty acids then reform into triglycerides.

Meanwhile, as these digestive "end products" leave the micelles and are absorbed into the villi, the micelles particles themselves are freed up to go back and absorb still more monoglycerides and fatty acids, and similarly transport them to the epithelial cell walls.

Thus, the bile acid micelles perform a ferrying function, which is essential to fat absorption.

Somebody really knew what they were doing when they put all this together, and how important it was!

Without bile salts, most of the lipids in food would be excreted in feces, undigested.

The resulting molecules are then moved along the small intestine to be absorbed into either the lymphatic system (long-chain fatty acids) or taken directly to the liver (short- and medium-chain fatty acids).

Consider that 30 percent of your fat, after it's digested, is water soluble. As such, it goes directly to the liver. The rest of it—and this includes the three essential fatty acids we covered earlier—is fat soluble and must go through the lymphatic system. Unless you exercise and breathe correctly, you're not going to be moving lymph very well. Where does the body put its toxins? In the lymphatic system. So all that sitting fat is just storing toxins.

Who has the most lymphatic trouble? Women. Who eats less protein and therefore generates less HCl production? Women.

The bottom line: If you're digesting protein well, you're going to have more stomach acid, first to digest that protein, and second because you're liberating acid when you break those protein bonds.

Now, who has most of the gallbladder trouble?

Women.

They teach it in the schools. It's called the 4F club: You're female, forty, fat and fertile, and you're going to have gallbladder trouble. And you're headed for lymphatic congestion. All of this stems from stomach acid deficiency, poor biliary flow, and eating too much sugar because you don't digest fat.

And so the biochemical wheel comes full circle.

Again, without bile, nothing moves forward.

Into The Liver

Here's where the final bit of magic comes in, made possible by two highly specialized enzyme forces.

Again, 30 percent of absorbed lipids are water soluble short- and medium-chain fatty acids and go to the liver immediately, while the other 70 percent are fat-soluble, long-chain fatty acids and have to make their way to the liver via the lymphatic system and the bloodstream.

Everything absorbed into the body through the intestine is contaminated—even after enzyme-packing white blood cells in the intestine have done their best to eliminate as many bacteria and toxins as possible. So once the short-chain fatty acids enter the liver, they go to the liver sinusoid, which is a waiting room where another line of lymphatic follicles finishes the cleansing job. The liver can now work on them.

Then there are the fat-soluble, long-chain fatty acids that have come to the liver by way of the lymphatics and the bloodstream. Before the liver can work on them, they must be made water soluble. This is where the first of two enzyme forces come into play, attaching an oxygen molecule to these fatty acids. This makes them water soluble.

And this is where the real drama begins. The biochemical process involved in converting these fatty acids from fat soluble to water soluble also creates free radicals, which are enormously toxic. These unstable molecules must be "quenched" immediately. This is the job of the second layer of enzymes. It's a critical process, and one that is entirely enzyme-driven.

And this is the critical point.

The quenching of free radicals is enzyme-driven and only enzyme-driven. It's not about vitamins A, B, C or E, or various vitamin/mineral combinations and everything else under the sun promoted as an antioxidant.

While they are widely used in dietary supplements and unabashedly promoted for their antioxidant powers, in preventing free-radical damage and everything from cancer to coronary heart disease, the large trials looking at myriad supplements, including beta-carotene, vitamins A and C, selenium, etc., in various combinations, have found no effect on any of the above, or mortality.

Chapter 6—Lipid: The Last Resort

Vitamins are co-enzymes. They have to be incorporated into the enzymes. They are only involved in preventing free radical damage when they are the co-enzyme part of the worker enzyme.

It's the enzymes that do the work. Without them, nothing gets done.

And when they're finished their antioxidant work, the liver does its own magic, and finally moves the end products to one of three places: into the blood, into the bile, and into the lymph, where it's all recirculated.

Talk about intelligent design!

Advertising Hype About Essential Amino Acids

Now's a good time to clear up some misinformation about fats.

First, approximately 40 percent to 45 percent of calories in the normal American diet are derived from fats, which is about equal to the calories derived from carbohydrates. This makes lipids as important as carbohydrates in providing the body with energy, despite all the flack they take.

Furthermore, much of the carbohydrate ingested with each meal is converted into lipids—i.e., triglycerides—and then stored in fat cells for later use as energy.

The only way the body can store energy is as fat.

There are two types of fat cells in the body—white cells and brown cells. Triglycerides are stored in the white fat cells. The brown cells secrete enzymes and molecules to burn up the triglycerides in the white fat cells as energy is needed.

On the issue of weight loss, while it may seem that eating a low-fat diet is a good way to lose weight, this is not necessarily true. The reason? The body is going to convert and store excess calories in the form of fat to meet increased energy needs as they arise, no matter what you do. This can lead to obesity and diabetes when brown cells cannot burn up stored fat fast enough.

High on the list of foods headed for fat storage are simple carbohydrates—breads, pastas, sugars, etc. These are the "bad carbohydrates," which are burned quickly for energy when eaten, or converted to fat and stored quickly. So if you're not running a mile, that cupcake you just ate is most likely headed for fat storage. Furthermore, people who are under chronic stress—i.e., structural, visceral, emotional—are much more likely to put on weight, because the body is constantly storing fat to meet energy needs.

The only way to lose weight in a healthy manner is by eating good carbohydrates—fresh fruits and vegetables, which contain their own enzymes and are burned slowly. This way you have a continual flow of energy, and the body never has to go to protein and fats for energy, and you don't have to store fat.

On the subject of magic bullets. There are none.

A doctor once approached me at a seminar I was giving, and asked me "What do I take for this?" My response: "If we put you and Beyoncé at the end of a long continuum, do you honestly think the two of you would fall into a national average that would make any sense for either one of you?" It can't be done. Not if you want to get sick people well. And yet, that is how nutrition is often practiced.

There is no magic bullet. Vitamin A, vitamin B, vitamin C, omega-3s and omega-6s are not the be-all and end-all they're hyped up to be. A health care provider would do better looking at each

Chapter 6—Lipid: The Last Resort

individual's energy deficiencies rather than applying a magic bullet formulated to fit a national average that does not exist.

> **Food *for* Thought**
>
> There are no average people. We are all individuals. You can have two patients with a particular disorder, and the approach to getting both of them well could be quite different. If you apply that national average, you stand a very good chance of getting neither of them well.

This makes even more sense when we consider that the energy deficiency is usually the first sign of trouble.

Vitamin and mineral deficiencies generally take 60 to 90 days to appear, symptomatically. Food enzyme deficiencies, as Howell noted, can take years. They appear as chronic degeneration, leading over time to chronic diseases like arthritis, cancer, heart disease and diabetes.

Energy deficiencies, on the other hand, show up in just hours. The body will normally take care of the problem without the person even knowing what's going on, as it shifts from burning carbohydrate to protein. This can't go on for long though, without becoming a major drain on one's energy checking account. And it can't use the plasma proteins, which are reserved for maintaining homeostasis. By the time the body shifts to burning stored fat, the problem has become aggravated into a chronic condition.

So where does the magic bullet fit into all of this? It doesn't.

And while certain vitamins and minerals have been promoted as magic bullets, with antioxidant powers to prevent all manner of diseases—from heart disease to diabetes and cancer—saturated fats, which are found in animal fat products, such as cream, cheese, butter and fatty meats, as well as coconut oil, cottonseed oil and chocolate, have been demonized and accused of causing all of the above.

The belief that saturated fat will increase your risk of heart disease and heart attacks is simply not true. In fact, when you eat, digest, absorb and use saturated fats, they slow down absorption so that you can go longer without feeling hungry, as well as provide a concentrated source of energy.

Saturated fatty acids are building blocks. They are used to make a variety of hormones and hormone-like substances, as well as cell membranes. They are also used for the conversion of carotene to vitamin A for mineral absorption, along with a host of other biological processes. And they act as carriers for fat-soluble vitamins A, D, E and K.

They lower cardiovascular risk. The addition of saturated fats to the diet has been shown to reduce the levels of lipoproteins in the blood. Research has also shown that when women diet, those who eat the greater percentage of the total fat in their diets as saturated fat, lose the most weight.

Saturated fats make for stronger bones. According to one of the foremost research experts in dietary fats and human health, there is a case to be made that saturated fats should make up 50 percent of the total fats in a person's diet. Why? Because they are required for calcium to be effectively incorporated into bone.

They protect the liver from alcohol and various medications, including acetaminophen and other medications used to treat pain and arthritis.

They are essential to healthy lung function. The fat content of the protective surfactant that coats the air spaces in the lungs is 100 percent saturated fatty acids.

The fact that saturated fatty acids are essential to good brain health is a no-brainer, given that the brain is mainly made of fat and cholesterol, and the lion's share of the fatty acids in the brain are saturated. A diet deficient in healthy saturated fats robs the brain of the raw materials it needs to function optimally.

Moreover, certain fatty acids, like those found in butter, lard, coconut oil and palm oil function directly as signaling messengers. They influence metabolism, including the appropriate release of insulin.

Then there's the role in maintaining a strong immune system.

Saturated fats found in butter and coconut oil (myristic acid and lauric acid) are useful as antiviral agents (caprylic acid), and can also be effective as anti-caries, anti-plaque, and anti-fungal agents (lauric acid). They are also useful in lowering cholesterol levels (palmitic and stearic acids). And as modulators of genetic regulation, they are useful in preventing cancer (butyric acid).

Finally, loss of sufficient saturated fatty acids in white blood cells hampers their ability to recognize and destroy foreign invaders, such as viruses, bacteria and fungi.

So that's the good word on the much maligned saturated fats.

Finally, when it comes to fats, it all boils down to the previously mentioned end product—the all-important prostaglandins. Which fatty acid breaks down to the highest-quality prostaglandin? That would be essential linolenic acid.

Basically, the body only looks at three types of fatty acids. Those are the three essential amino acids—linolenic, linoleic and arachadonic. Those three are absolutely fundamental. They are as fundamental as amino acids are in the protein chain.

Omega-3s and omega-6s, for all the hype they get, are not fundamental. They are way down the chain in terms of importance, and they breakdown at best to moderately effective prostaglandins.

So much for magic bullets.

> **At the end of the day, it all comes back to Howell—to enzymes. If the enzymes aren't there to do the work—salivary lipase, gastric lipase and food enzymes in the stomach, pancreatic lipase in the duodenum, and the enzymes that convert fat-soluble fatty acids to water soluble and quench the resulting free radicals in the liver—it would be difficult, if not impossible, to enjoy a healthy life for very long.**

It's that simple.

Come up with one enzyme that will do all that—for everyone—and you've got your magic bullet.

In the meantime, the human body struggles along, with its compromised digestive system working to overcome the ill effects of an enzyme-deficient, cooked and processed diet that contributes nothing in the way of predigestion and breeds energy deficiencies like Halloween breeds ghosts on every street corner, looking for a sweet treat to quench their sugar craving.

An entire aspect of the predigestive process has been lost.

Chapter 6—Lipid: The Last Resort

> **Food *for* Thought**
>
> **But if you can identify the organ or organ system that is running on empty, and if you can deliver the nutrition it needs by way of an enzyme formula designed to digest those nutritional elements—carbohydrate, protein and/or fat—to an absorbable state, then you've given the body the energy it needs to heal itself.**

Epilogue

A Final Word

When Anthony Collier first came to my office in 1980, the National Enzyme Company (NEC), was pretty much the only game in town. Prior to Collier's taking it over in 1978, the house that Howell built in 1932 had remained a mere mom-and-pop mail-order operation. By the time I put in my five investigative years and began lecturing, in 1985, there still wasn't a food enzyme marketplace to speak of.

Little attention was being paid to food enzymes.

By 1993, however, when I formed my own company, Collier's NEC had become a worldwide operation, and the marketplace was filled with companies extolling the virtues of their enzyme formulas. Had he still been around, Doc Howell himself would have been stunned, and I suspect somewhat bewildered.

The Enzyme Advantage

It is impossible to predict the future that food enzymes will have in the healing arts. However, one thing is certain. While the removal of naturally occurring food enzymes from our diet is necessary to achieve greater shelf life, in order to feed an ever-increasing world population, this progress comes at a price. Dr. Howell first observed this back in the 1920s.

The need for food enzymes to perform their predigestive duties, as Nature originally intended, can be understood in their absence—an increasingly compromised digestive system, which has become a breeding ground for degenerative diseases. It follows that adding food enzyme supplements to an individual's dietary routine can restore predigestion and be an overall benefit to health.

But it doesn't stop there.

The plethora of food enzyme products available to consumers today is welcome, of course. But for those seeking relief from nagging health problems not yet diagnosed as disease, these commercial formulas, while helpful, may not resolve the problem.

Once again, the "one size fits all" concept simply does not apply in health care.

The key is in the use of inductive rather than deductive reasoning, and applying that reasoning to diagnosis and treatment.

For example, instead of simply reaching for the aspirin at the onset of yet another headache, providers should ask themselves, what is the cause of this headache? Is it the result of emotional stress, or perhaps working too hard and not getting enough rest? Or is it caused by diet, overconsumption, or inadequate digestion? Could it be related to poor bowel elimination? Is there a structural issue resulting in increased involuntary muscle contraction?

Epilogue—A Final Word

One thing is certain. If we continuously reach for the over-the-counter quick fix, the cause of the headache or headaches may remain unabated. Unless it is resolved, the problem will progress and possibly lead to a chronic degenerative process. This unequivocal statement brings us back to Dr. Edward Howell, whose life work inspired the writing of this book.

Indeed, enzymes are Nature's workers. And food enzymes are essential to a healthy digestive system and adequate delivery of nutrition to the body's organs.

Beyond this, however, if inductive methods are used to diagnose where a person's energy deficiency is and what is needed in the way of nutrition to resolve this deficiency, then food enzyme supplements can be used to deliver that nutrition to the struggling organ system to restore normal function and maintain health.

That is the vital message of this book.

H. Loomis

Selected Bibliography

Introduction

Feinstein, Alvin. *Clinical Judgment.* The Williams & Wilkins Co., 1967

Monk's Roll: Lives of the Fellows of the Royal College of Physicians of London, Vol III (18-1-1825). London: RCP, p. 205. 1878.

Chapter 1

Allison, Anthony. "Lysosomes and Disease." *Scientific American,* November 1967.

Howell, Edward, *Enzyme Nutrition.* Avery Publishing Group, p. 1-13. 1985.

Howell, Edward. *Food Enzymes for Health and Longevity,* Second Edition, Lotus Press, p. 8. March 1994.

Kouchakoff, P. The influence of food cooking on the blood formula of man. *Proceedings: First International Congress of Microbiology.* Paris. 1930.

Chapter 2

Five Dimensions of Co-Intelligence. Accessed at www.co-intelligence.org/I-5dimensions.html

Palmer, D.D. *The Chiropractic Adjuster.* Portland Printing House, 1910.

Selye, Hans. *The Stress of Life.* New York, McGraw-Hill Book Company, Inc. 1956.

Waterson, David. "Sir James MacKenzie and the Sympathetic Innervation of Striated Muscle." *British Medical Journal.* March 7; 1(3349): p. 482. 1925. Accessed at http://www.ncbi.nlm.nih.gov/pmc/articles/PMC2226510/.

Chapter 3

Howell, Edward. *Enzyme Nutrition.* Garden City, NY: Avery Publishing Group. Chapter 1. 1985.

Howell, Edward. *Food Enzymes for Health and Longevity,* Twin Lakes, WI: Lotus Press, p. 8. 1994.

Chapter 4

Cooper, Edward C. "A Common Ankyrin-G-Based Mechanism Retains KCNQ and NaV Channels at Electrically Active Domains of the Axon." *Journal of Neuroscience.* 26(10):2599-2613. August 2006.

Selected Bibliography

Chapter 5

Romans S, Clarkson R, Einstein G, Petrovic M, Stewart D., "Mood and the menstrual cycle: a review of prospective data studies," *Gend Med.*; 9(5):361-384. October 2012.

Mayo Clinic on PMS: Accessed at http://www.mayoclinic.org/diseases-conditions/premenstrual-syndrome/basics/causes/con-20020003

Los Angeles Times. "Woman dies after being in water-drinking contest," January 14, 2007. (Associated Press). Accessed at http://www.nbcnews.com/id/16614865/ns/us_news-life/t/woman-dies-after-water-drinking-contest/#.VSVhCE10zEY.

Chapter 6

Cleghorn, Geoffrey J.; Shepherd, Ross W. *Cystic fibrosis: nutritional and intestinal disorders.* Boca Raton, FL: CRC Press. 1989.

Index

A

ACTH 101

active ingredient 53

Acupuncture 54, 55

alcohol 73, 161

allopathic 1

alternative 5, 9

amino acids 51, 92, 93, 100, 116, 120, 121, 122, 127, 128, 133, 136, 162

amylase 10, 51, 69, 76, 85, 104, 107, 108, 109, 143

ancient healing systems 52

anxiety 9, 96, 110, 114, 115, 133

arthritis 9, 11, 16, 68, 101, 159, 161

asthma 101

Ayurveda 52, 53

B

bear 96

bile 5, 21, 44, 53, 60, 78, 99, 136, 149, 150, 151, 152, 153, 154, 155, 157

biochemical 5, 91, 93, 97, 114, 155, 156

blood 8, 9, 22, 24, 28, 29, 30, 31, 33, 42, 43, 44, 46, 49, 50, 52, 59, 60, 68, 69, 71, 72, 73, 81, 82, 83, 84, 87, 95, 97, 98, 99, 100, 101, 109, 116, 119, 122, 123, 124, 128, 130, 132, 133, 135, 144, 146, 147, 149, 156, 157, 160, 161, 167

blood platelets 59, 146

"blood thinners" 99

brain 36, 37, 39, 42, 43, 45, 51, 84, 87, 88, 93, 95, 96, 99, 100, 105, 107, 110, 111, 114, 119, 122, 124, 126, 144, 161

Buffy Coat Analysis 59

C

Cannon, Walter B. 40

carbohydrate 20, 70, 87, 88, 92, 93, 101, 102, 103, 104, 105, 106, 107, 109, 111, 120, 142, 143, 144, 145, 157, 159

carbohydrate deficiency 102, 105, 106, 107, 142

carcinogenic 103

caregiver 97, 98

cells 10, 11, 28, 29, 33, 39, 40, 41, 42, 43, 46, 49, 50, 59, 60, 61, 65, 68, 69, 70, 71, 72, 83, 84, 85, 91, 92, 93, 98, 100, 102, 103, 105, 116, 119, 122, 123, 124, 126, 144, 146, 147, 150, 156, 157, 158, 161

cellulase 10, 30, 51, 76, 79, 81, 85, 103

cellulose 78, 79, 103

Chinese medicine 54, 55

chiropractor 18, 26, 27, 37, 38, 48, 75, 93, 99, 131, 135

cholecystokinin 69

cholesterol 41, 99, 133, 161

chronic 9, 16, 17, 26, 29, 38, 52, 66, 73, 77, 87, 91, 93, 94, 96, 97, 98, 99, 100, 101, 119, 123, 131, 132, 141, 158, 159, 160, 165

chronic diseases 16, 17, 159

circulating immune complexes 72

circulation 52, 72, 132

co-enzyme 157

common denominator 31, 52, 54, 55, 61

constipation 44, 70, 79, 96, 105, 106

contractions 38, 46, 55, 74, 77, 78, 83, 84, 88, 93, 94, 98, 99, 107, 108, 109, 129, 130, 143, 144

cooked and processed food 16

cortisone 101

D

dehydration 106

dermatomes 37

diarrhea 70, 79, 80, 105

diet 8, 16, 17, 54, 58, 60, 61, 68, 74, 78, 80, 81, 82, 86, 94, 95, 101, 102, 104, 105, 106, 111, 117, 120, 134, 145, 148, 152, 153, 157, 158, 160, 161, 164

dietary fats 142, 149, 150, 160

dietary fiber 102

digestion 5, 10, 11, 16, 17, 21, 28, 29, 30, 31, 32, 41, 53, 57, 60, 67, 68, 69, 70, 71, 75, 76, 78, 79, 82, 94, 104, 105, 109, 117, 118, 132, 135, 140, 141, 149, 150, 151, 152, 164

Doshas 53

duodenum 50, 69, 150, 151

E

ectoderm 36, 53

embryonic layers 36

endocrine system 42, 143

endoderm 36, 53

energy 11, 40, 41, 42, 53, 54, 55, 58, 59, 60, 65, 69, 71, 74, 78, 79, 82, 84, 87, 88, 91, 92, 93, 94, 95, 96, 97, 98, 99, 100, 101, 102, 103, 104, 105, 106, 109, 110, 114, 116, 123, 125, 126, 130, 131, 132, 141, 143, 144, 157, 158, 159, 160, 165

energy bank account 100

enzyme deficiencies 30, 159

enzyme-deficient diet 58, 68, 74, 95

enzyme supplementation 94, 140

epiphany 35

equilibrium 49, 57

extracellular fluid 2, 40, 42, 86, 116

F

fatigue 38, 93, 106, 114, 130

fatty acids 91, 103, 120, 142, 145, 146, 148, 149, 150, 153, 154, 155, 156, 160, 161, 162

"fight or flight" 92, 141

flora 70

food 6, 3, 10, 11, 16, 17, 29, 31, 40, 41, 43, 50, 54, 57, 58, 63, 65, 66, 67, 68, 69, 70, 71, 72, 73, 74, 75, 76, 78, 79, 80, 82, 83, 92, 94, 103, 114, 115, 117, 128, 129, 135, 148, 149, 150, 151, 152, 154, 163, 164, 165, 167

Food Enzyme Concept 16

Food enzyme deficiencies 159

fruits 10, 78, 80, 81, 101, 102, 103, 104, 105, 121, 158

G

galactose 79, 104

gas 44, 70, 79, 80, 96, 103, 105

gastrointestinal tract 70, 71, 146

general adaptation syndrome 45, 97

glucose 79, 84, 87, 92, 93, 96, 97, 99, 100, 101, 103, 104, 105, 106, 107, 109, 110, 116, 131, 144

glycerol 150

glycogen 92, 99, 100, 101, 104, 107

H

health 6, 1, 2, 3, 9, 11, 15, 17, 34, 45, 46, 52, 53, 54, 57, 61, 64, 68, 74, 75, 78, 93, 96, 103, 107, 115, 118, 121, 127, 128, 129, 141, 149, 159, 160, 161, 164, 165

health care providers 6, 15, 64, 74, 93

heartburn 96, 135

heart rate 41, 97

heat kills 16

Head, Henry 37

herbs 53, 54, 85, 92, 140, 143

Hippocrates 9, 56, 58, 59

holistic 140

holistic treatments 140

Holy Grail 5, 64

homeostasis 2, 3, 38, 40, 41, 42, 43, 44, 46, 47, 49, 51, 52, 53, 57, 60, 61, 64, 65, 74, 86, 91, 95, 98, 99, 104, 116, 121, 122, 123, 124, 125, 126, 128, 131, 137, 141, 160

Howell, Edward 10, 16, 65, 165

hormonal organs 141

hydrochloric acid (HCl) 43, 69

hypoflexia 60

I

imbalance 53, 95, 135, 136

indican 71

indigestion 96, 135

inflammation 27, 33, 49, 72, 101, 146

Insoluble fiber 102

internal environment 40, 41

Intolerance 109

intracellular fluid 40

in vitro fertilization 140

involuntary muscle contractions 38, 46, 74, 77, 83, 84, 93, 94, 98, 99, 107, 108, 109, 129, 143, 144

iron deficiency 50

J

jejunum 80, 104

K

kidneys 103, 124, 132

Knee flexion 47

L

lactose 79, 80, 104, 105, 109

large intestine 55, 70, 71

"leaky gut" syndrome 71

leukocytes 72, 146

lipase 10, 30, 31, 51, 69, 76, 85, 136, 143, 149, 150, 151, 153, 154

lipid deficiency 84, 87, 142, 144, 145

lipids 10, 84, 85, 93, 120, 135, 141, 142, 143, 144, 145, 153, 154, 155, 157

M

MacKenzie, James 37, 168

magic bullet 5, 10, 159, 160

marshmallow root 92

melancholy 56, 60

mesoderm 36, 53

metabolic enzymes 134

"missing link" 65

motor reflexes 38

mucosal lining 152

muscle tension headaches 93

N

neurological innervations 94

neurons 37

nutrients 40, 42, 45, 46, 53, 54, 58, 68, 69, 70, 74, 91, 94, 104, 105, 123, 124, 125, 130, 131, 133, 145

nutrition 6, 8, 11, 45, 46, 47, 57, 61, 63, 65, 75, 78, 81, 86, 91, 94, 95, 98, 101, 115, 120, 126, 130, 131, 135, 136, 144, 145, 158, 165

O

okra 92

organ system 11, 18, 54, 61, 63, 65, 165

ovotarians 127

P

pancreas 16, 38, 42, 50, 68, 69, 70, 76, 77, 78, 80, 150

pancreatic amylase 104

pancreatic enzymes 17, 21, 77

parasympathetic 52, 95

parotid glands 69

pathogens 70

pepsin 5, 17, 44, 69, 150

pepsinogen 5, 44, 69, 150

pH 41, 42, 44, 117, 123, 149, 150

phlegmatic 56, 60

pituitary gland 42, 141

plasma proteins 42, 121, 123, 124, 125, 159

potassium 43, 58, 60, 70, 92, 95, 101, 105, 107, 134

prostaglandin 148, 162

protease 10, 16, 30, 31, 32, 33, 34, 35, 49, 51, 69, 76, 83, 85, 111, 118, 143

Protein 11, 42, 43, 58, 60, 113, 120, 122, 125, 132, 133

protomorphogens 50

putrefaction 16, 71

pyloric valve 69

R

receptors 36

reduction 140

reflexes 38

reproductive system 99, 100, 144

respiration 45

Reston, James 4

Rouleaux 50

S

Selye, Hans 8, 44, 97

Shakespeare 56

shelf life 66, 68, 79, 94, 164

shingles 37

shoulder blades 93, 94, 119, 132

slippery elm 92

small intestine 17, 55, 69, 70, 71, 79, 104, 149, 151, 152, 153, 154

soluble fiber 103

Sophocles 56

spinal cord 36, 37

starch 69, 102, 103, 104, 107

stimulus stress 45

stomach acid 5, 43, 104, 119, 149, 151, 152, 153, 155

stress 2, 8, 17, 18, 20, 21, 28, 31, 35, 36, 37, 38, 43, 44, 45, 46, 47, 48, 50, 55, 63, 77, 84, 87, 91, 93, 94, 97, 98, 99, 100, 101, 109, 110, 122, 126, 131, 140, 141, 143, 148, 158, 164

Stress of Life, The 8, 44, 168

Stress Without Distress 44

stroke 7

sublingual glands 69

submandibular glands 69

sucrose 79, 104, 105

sugar 29, 41, 60, 73, 79, 101, 104, 105, 106, 107, 109, 110, 111, 120, 131, 155

sympathetic 52, 95, 96, 97, 144

symptoms 2, 8, 9, 10, 15, 18, 19, 20, 22, 23, 28, 35, 37, 46, 47, 49, 50, 51, 60, 61, 64, 74, 75, 80, 86, 87, 88, 95, 96, 97, 98, 99, 100, 101, 103, 106, 107, 109, 110, 111, 113, 114, 115, 117, 118, 128, 131, 133, 134, 136, 142, 143, 144, 145, 152, 153

T

thyroid 42, 98, 99, 141

thyroxine 98, 122

U

Unani-Tibb 56, 57, 58

universal intelligence 38, 39, 43, 51, 52

urinalysis 2, 9, 22, 30, 32, 49, 59, 78, 81, 84, 115, 117

V

vegetarian 127

viscera 38

visceral 17, 18, 20, 22, 35, 36, 37, 38, 48, 49, 50, 61, 74, 86, 87, 88, 91, 93, 99, 107, 126, 129, 131, 132, 158

vitamins 10, 20, 21, 22, 50, 58, 61, 67, 70, 82, 85, 92, 101, 102, 105, 106, 134, 149, 153, 156, 160

voluntary contractions 38

W

waste removal 40, 46, 98, 106

Wolff, Caspar Friedrich 36

XYZ

X-ray 50, 129

About the Authors

Howard F. Loomis, Jr., D.C., F.I.A.C.A., is a 1967 graduate of Logan Chiropractic College. Dr. Loomis's interest in nutritional food enzymes began when he had the privilege of working with Edward Howell, M.D., the food enzyme pioneer.

He has taught his system to professional health care practitioners since 1985. As founder and president of The Loomis Institute™ of Enzyme Nutrition, he has forged a remarkable career as an educator, having conducted countless seminars in the United States, Canada, Germany, and New Zealand on the clinical identification of food enzyme deficiencies.

He has extensive background in enzymes and enzyme formulations. He is currently president of his own enzyme company, Enzyme Formulations®, Inc. With his exciting approach to health and wellness, Dr. Loomis is now preparing others to take health care into the next century.

Arnold Mann has been writing about medicine for 30 years. His cover stories for *TIME* and *USA Weekend Magazine* have earned him recognition as one of the nation's leading medical journalists. Mr. Mann served as co-author of Dr. Keith Black's book, *Brain Surgeon: A Doctor's Inspiring Encounters with Mortality and Miracles* (Grand Central Publishing, 2010), which was nominated for an NAACP Image Award (Best Nonfiction Book).

Mr. Mann has also written extensively for publications of the National Institutes of Health. He served as personal writer for the Director of the National Cancer Institute, and he oversaw publication of the Institute's *Annual Progress Report to Congress.*

Made in the USA
Middletown, DE
02 December 2015